T0246286

BADASS BONITA

BADASS BONITA

Break the Silence,
Become a Revolution,
Unearth Your Inner Guerrera

KIM GUERRA, MFT

balance

New York   Boston

Copyright © 2024 by Kimberly Guerra

Cover design by Jim Datz

Cover art by Victoria Villasana

Cover copyright © 2024 by Hachette Book Group, Inc.

Balance

Hachette Book Group

1290 Avenue of the Americas

New York, NY 10104

GCP-Balance.com

@GCPBalance

First Edition: September 2024

Balance is an imprint of Grand Central Publishing. The Balance name and logo are registered trademarks of Hachette Book Group, Inc.

The publisher is not responsible for websites (or their content) that are not owned by the publisher.

Balance books may be purchased in bulk for business, educational, or promotional use. For information, please contact your local bookseller or the Hachette Book Group Special Markets Department at special.markets@hbgusa.com.

Print book interior design by Bart Dawson

Library of Congress Cataloging-in-Publication Data has been applied for.

ISBNs: 9781538742433 (hardcover), 9781538742457 (ebook)

Printed in the United States of America

LSC-C

Printing 1, 2024

This is for the niñas who are now mujeres
learning to love themselves

CONTENTS

PART IV: USING YOUR WINGS

BADASS
BONITA

INTRODUCTION

B adass Bonita was born out of a need for self-love and commu-
nity. Badass Bonitas are the ones who are no longer willing to
stay calladitas. We are the ones who are ready to give ourselves wings.
I didn't always have wings. Sometimes it feels like I am still trying
them on. Like a new pair of huaraches, you have to walk in them
for a while para que la piel se acostumbre a tus pies. This is how I felt
about using my voice. Each step is a victory in itself. These words will
tell you about the victories, metamorphosis, and paths that led me to
my voice. May the words in this book serve as a guide for you to find
your own voice and use it.

Some of these paths were assigned to me from before I was born.
These were the paths I walked because mi mami walked in them, and
she walked because her mami walked in them. They hold their own
stories in their huaraches and wings. Somos guerreras full of victo-
ries and battle wounds. I've touched their scars. I've felt their huara-
ches on my ass. Their paths are intertwined with mine. We form an
intergenerational trenza with our stories.

After years of going through therapy myself and becoming a
licensed marriage and family therapist, I am a firm believer in my
voice's ability to give me wings. As a survivor of childhood sexual

abuse, the eldest daughter of a Latin Pentecostal family, and someone who grew up without a positive father figure, I spent most of my life seeking approval. I was the first in my family to graduate from high school and college. A week after my graduation from Cornell University, I got married to the white, cis-het Norwegian president of my Christian club. I continued to check the boxes of what a good Christian woman should and shouldn't be.

I was living in Seattle in a sea of white people, feeling out of place and lost, and desperately missing the Latine community I grew up with.

Memories of my childhood always included hearing the water running in my mother's bath. She would take baths en la madrugada because it was the only time she had for herself. As I grew up, I followed in her footsteps. During one of my baths, an existential crisis ensued. I felt like I was going to die. Surrounded by water, I could feel the fire inside myself fading. I was becoming a whisper of myself. Years of taking care of others while neglecting myself had left me feeling empty and like I had nothing left to give. I had two choices: perish or choose myself. I am here. I chose me. In this particular 4:00 a.m. bath, three words came to me: "Brown Badass Bonita."

They were a reclamation of my power and identity. They gave me fuerza and hope. They reminded me I was the one that had decided to heal, the one that had decided to break generational patterns, and the one that had decided to finally say: "Fuck being a calladita." I could feel these were life-changing words. I wanted to wear them like a statement and a shield. I designed a T-shirt with them superimposed on a picture of bougainvilleas, the colorful flower petals reminding me of my homes: Los Angeles and Mexico. When it finally came in the mail, I put the T-shirt on, took a picture, and posted it on Instagram.

It blew up.

Messages from women all over the world filled my inbox, saying they were also Brown Badass Bonitas, pero no one had ever told them that before. They wanted to buy the shirt. At that point, there was only one Brown Badass Bonita shirt in the world: mine.

Soon, I opened an Etsy shop and sent links to each person that wanted to get their hands on their own Brown Badass Bonita T-shirt. I sold one hundred of them the first weekend, including handwritten notes in each order. My community was finding me. In that moment, I realized I was not only fighting for me, but for—and with—us all. In that moment, I knew I wasn't alone. No estamos solas.

A few weeks after the initial launch of Brown Badass Bonita, I decided to host the first ever Brown Badass Bonita meetup. I turned on my FBI mode and reached out to whoever I could find that could possibly be Latina in Seattle. I sent out messages and emails to random women and people with Latina-sounding names, inviting them to bring their art, music, and their whole selves to the event. When the time came, sixty people gathered at a little local park. We ate the tamales my best friend Edwin and I had made early that morning. We talked and made friendships that still stand to this day. Strangers turned into family. Cómplices en el rescate de nosotras mismas. I couldn't believe it. The audacity. The absolute beauty. This is what being a Badass Bonita is all about.

I began sharing my writing and healing journey with this community of Badass Bonitas through my poems, posts, art, and events. At the time, I was getting my master's degree in marriage and family therapy. I was also getting a divorce. After the divorce, I felt like I had a second chance, and I began saying yes to the things I had said no to out of fear. This included turning my poems into a book, *Mariposa*, and becoming a writer. I went on a tour after *Mariposa* made some bestseller lists and I felt the power of our community as I met with Badass Bonitas across the country. Our journey was just beginning.

Now, as a marriage and family therapist, I see how important and healing it is for us to embark on this journey of revolutionary self-love and collective liberation together. We heal in community. Many of us grew up hearing therapy was for the gringos and locos. It was not meant for people like us. The therapists didn't look, speak, or live like us, and their spaces didn't seem to invite people like us. Pero now, we are creating those bridges and tables so we may have access to spaces where we can heal. We have—and we are—the medicine.

This book is for those mujeres who are ready to build and cross bridges. This book is for the women coming across healing work for the first time, for the women who started their journey to self-love and hit a wall, for the women who know they need to take care of themselves but nobody taught them how, for queer women, for mothers, for creatives, and for the ones who want to be soft. This book is for the mijas, tías, madrinas, and abuelas. For strong women and for those who are tired of having to be so strong. I write for mujeres like you and me.

I am honored to be a guide on your journey, a bridge to a healing version of yourself. I want to offer what I've learned in my own journey. I'd like to share with you the things I wish I knew then and walk alongside you the way I needed someone to walk alongside me. When I first made the choice to love myself, I had no idea how to actually do it. I just knew I wanted and needed it—desperately. After reading a nayyirah waheed poem, I began asking myself one simple question: How will I love myself today? This little question changed my whole life. It taught me that self-love truly is a revolution.

The revolution looked different every day. It looked like: Today, I love myself enough to do things that bring me joy. Today, I refuse to silence myself, to embrace healing through therapy and leave this unhealthy marriage. Today, loving myself looks like saying, "Me vale" to las tías criticonas.

I ask you the same question:

How will you love yourself today?

If you don't know the answer yet, it's okay. The term self-love has become somewhat diluted with overuse. I will not attempt to define it because it is not a one-size-fits-all kind of concept. Self-love looks and feels different for each person. This book will help you get to a place where you define it for yourself. You choose how you will love yourself. You will then witness how this self-love will transform your life. Not me. You. Tú. Tu corazón dispuesto a amarse, sanarse y liberarse. That is what makes it so powerful, so sacred. Living in active and intentional liberation requires us to embrace our identity and believe that what we have to say is important because who we are is important not only for us but for the generations that come after us. Self-love is the gold that weaves us back together and carries the metamorphosis forward. Self-love is the beginning of your revolution, and it remains an ongoing catalyst toward liberation.

Mujer, I am going to be real with you: being a Badass Bonita is something you are born with and something that you choose. It is the choice to do and be whoever the fuck you want. Es la decisión de vivir en paz. It means making the conscious decision to choose what love looks like to you. Love can be the ability to look back at your past selves with compassion, to look at your present self con ojos de amor, and to commit to the mujer you are becoming. I set boundaries, wrote a book of poems, started a business, and welcomed healing into my life—all as an answer to that question. I will love myself enough to say, "Fuck being calladita."

To be a badass, you must stop shrinking. You must stop seeing yourself as less than. You must love yourself.

If someone you care about is bleeding, you'll help them heal the wound so the bleeding stops, ¿sí o no? Claro que sí. It is now time to do that for yourself. Love yourself enough to do whatever it takes to heal your bleeding wounds. Es tiempo de sanar. To do this, we need to not only identify the unhealed wounds, but we must also find the source of the wounds—la raíz de las heridas. The source of our wounds and the medicine often lead us back to our mothers and grandmothers, and the many that came before them. Their wounds are often rooted in a culture and society that perpetuated trauma and oppression. We will transform the trauma through this work. You are the medicine and the mariposa.

These pages are intended to guide you through a metamorphosis from calladita to mujer mariposa. Together, we will walk through the four stages of your transformation, and I'll be here to accompany you through the process of learning, unlearning, and healing. The journey will look like this:

PART I: THE CATERPILLAR

Our stories begin in the womb. We are connected to our ancestors: their wounds, their prayers, their stories. They did the best they could with what they had. In order to understand this fully, we must understand the stories, messages, and systems established before us in order to see their impact on our lives and the roles we play within the system we were born into. This part will focus on assessing the

Introduction xvii

soil in which we were planted and unearthing deep-rooted values and messages woven into our DNA.

PART II: THE CHRYSALIS

We begin investigating the messages that took root as you developed your identity and began navigating your place in this world. This is the stage where we begin receiving messages like "Calladita te ves más bonita," which inform us about who and how we "should" be. This is also the stage in which many of us encounter abuse, trauma, and systems of oppression. We in turn internalize the oppressive messages and use them to cultivate our sense of self. This part will focus on identifying the framework and messages which contributed to our wounds, relational patterns, and identity development.

PART III: THE BREAKTHROUGH

You were born and created to become the most powerful, beautiful, liberated version of yourself—it is in your DNA. Tienes todo lo que necesitas para sanar y transformar tu vida. You have all you need to heal and transform your life. It is time to identify the places you are hurting—the reason you've kept quiet—and begin the healing process. This is the hardest part. The chrysalis stage is the place in which we go inward and the undoing begins. In order to heal, we must let go of the messages and shame which keep us from believing we are worthy of love. We must unsubscribe to the lie that our voice isn't important. This is where we unlearn, undo, cry ugly, and choose to heal because we are tired of being calladitas. You will learn to navigate from the chrysalis stage of healing (identifying wounds and entering into the shadow work necessary to develop wings) to the breakthrough (breaking free of the cycles and out of the old frameworks that were keeping you from flying).

PART IV: USING YOUR WINGS

We shed the old self and emerge as a winged creature no longer weighed down and no longer calladita. Self-love is the gold that weaves us back together and carries the metamorphosis forward. Self-love is the beginning of your revolution, and it remains an ongoing catalyst toward liberation. It is time we learn how to use our wings. Living in active and intentional liberation requires us to embrace our identity and believe that what we have to say is important because who we are is important not only for us, but for the generations that come after us. This part focuses on the significance of self-love, of stepping into a liberated lifestyle, and of passing on intergenerational healing. ¡A volar se ha dicho, mujer mariposa!

I write for mujeres who are ready to fight for their wings. This book is for guerreras fighting fear, shame, and silence. I warn you desde ahorita: se vale llorar. ¡Se vale gritar! Se vale hacer lo que te dé la chingada gana. One of my hopes for you is that by the time you finish reading this book you will no longer believe your worth is tied to your silence. I hope you become familiar with yourself, your wounds, and your power. Quiero que sepas que tienes—y eres—la medicina. You will know how badass and beautiful you are.

I am a firm believer that every revolution starts from within. Every wildfire starts with a tiny, somewhat unsuspecting spark, like the smallest decision to do something differently, or the slightest shift to welcome vulnerability and change. Your fire can start today. Porque todo esto es una decisión. We didn't choose the soil we were born into, but we can choose the garden we will plant. Ahí está la revolución. Y ahí empezaremos.

You are most beautiful when you love yourself, mujer mariposa. Your voice is powerful and necessary. What you have to say is important, because who you are is important. Calladita no te ves más bonita. Fuck that. ¡Usa tu voz, mija!

PART I

THE
CATERPILLAR

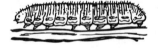

Chapter 1

The Soil You're Born Into

My mother gave birth to a winged creature
She looked at me
Unsure of how she could give birth to
something so strange
No one told her she also had wings
She spent her whole life believing
She was earthbound
Until she saw her daughter fly.

I magine if your mami knew she had wings. Many of us were niñas raised by mamis who didn't know they could fly. We are now mujeres giving ourselves wings. Quiero que este libro te apapache el corazón. Que llegue a las profundidades de tu alma. No por las palabras, ni por el contenido, sino por tu disponibilidad de amarte a ti misma. Quiero que este libro te inspire a ser el amor de tu vida, a darte alas y a gritar lo que siempre callaste. Te convertirás en una revolución viva, en una mujer que se dio alas.

A mi abuela le decían La Loba, the she-wolf. Her name is María Lourdes, which means she who bites. Her last name is Reyes. She who bites kings—that's mi Tita. She earned her Loba nickname because she was always ready to fight and she'd fight until she drew blood—it didn't matter if it was a man or a woman. Ella no se dejaba. Hasta que les veía sangre, she always told me. "I had no one to defend me, so I had to defend myself." Her father was a farmworker in California and would leave for months at a time. "He'd only come home to get my mom pregnant," she'd always say. Her mother was occupied with being the town seamstress and mother to eleven, of which mi Tita was the second-oldest daughter and a rainbow baby. My great-grandmother had a miscarriage before her and used the same name. From a young age, mi tita believed her mother named her the same because she wanted her to die too.

Mi Abue (great-grandmother) and mi Tita never had a good relationship. My grandmother was too wild. My great-grandmother was too heartbroken and angry to embrace a daughter como La Loba. Mi Abue, Josefina Villaseñor Pérez, was in love with another man when my great-grandfather la robó. This was a common practice back then, which translates quite accurately to kidnapping. The men would see a girl they liked (young virgins) and would take them as their wives just like that. This usually involved rape, as most of these girls did not know said "husband" nor did they consent to this "marriage"—love was irrelevant. Josefina was heartbroken. She had a boyfriend she wanted to marry, but after Alfredo (my great-grandfather) took her and raped her she was damaged goods. She tried returning to her family, but they wouldn't take her back. In order to preserve the family's honor, they forced her to marry Alfredo. Josefina hated him most of her life. She had little capacity to love the eleven children she bore for him. For her, it was a good thing he was gone most of the year en el campo. Although, whenever he came back, she was sure to get pregnant again. With each additional child, mi Abue lost more and more of herself. Su corazón se marchitó.

La Loba grew up believing she was unlovable and a source of shame to her family. She was raised with a mami con un corazón marchitado, un corazón que ya no podía dar amor. Although she spent her whole life chasing after it, she never got her mother's approval. Instead, her mother made sure to remind her, and the whole town, what a disappointment she was. Once over a lunch date, mi Tita told me her mother called her a puta in front of everyone at church. My grandmother had tears in her eyes as she spoke of her mother. Tita said, "Le tenía tanta rabia…me costó (y todavía me cuesta) mucho perdonarla. Sentí que mi vida era un fracaso. Sacrifiqué todo para ayudar a todos, y aun así nadie me aceptó." My grandmother inherited my great-grandmother's shame, pain, internalized machismo, racism, and homophobia. She passed most of this onto her daughter, mi mami. Mi Tita did her best to forgive and love despite not having received much, if any, love herself. She'd watch YouTube videos on forgiveness and aligning her chakras. She even joined WhatsApp groups for señoras who wanted to heal. Even so, she could only do so much with what little love she was given.

Beatriz Noemi means she who brings joy and pleasantness. Her last name is Guerra, war. A contradiction. My great-grandmother raised her with love and tenderness. Her own mother was absent, and always angry. My mother first heard "Calladita te ves más bonita" from the women who raised her (Abue y sus tías). They would tell her to stay quiet and never talk back to mi Tita. If my mom spoke up, mi Tita would beat her with her hands, cables, hangers, and whatever was nearby. Silence was my mother's key to survival. Her silence was her shield against my grandmother's physical and emotional abuse.

Mi Tita projected her rage and pain unto my mother. Her words hurt my mom the most. They lasted longer than the bruises on her pale skin. "Me hizo creer que nadie me quería y que yo le estorbaba a todos," she said. Mi mami spent her whole life trying to please everyone and be the best girl so they would love her. She had to earn her place, and maybe then she would be worthy of love. Mi Tita would make sure her daughter knew she was a burden. Mi mami, just like her mami and her mami's mami, grew up longing for her mami's love and acceptance. To this day, the longing remains.

La Loba just wanted to escape: correr y correr until she couldn't run any longer. She gave birth to Mimi, my mother, a little girl who grew up seeing her mother run and howl at the moon. Mimi became a teen mom the year after she stopped playing with Barbies. A woman who only wanted one thing: someone who loved her enough to stay. She gave birth to a mariposa who didn't know how to stay. La Loba's daughter gave birth to a winged creature.

I am the winged creature, and I, too, long for mi mami. I look at my hands and I see my mother, mi Tita, mi Abue. I feel the wounds that never healed. They are still bleeding. I'm fighting the wars they lost. I benefit from the blessings they fought and bled for. Because of their tears, I am able to fly. Because of their silence, yo no me voy a callar.

De mi abuela heredé las ganas de aullar. Pero en vez de sacar sangre, yo quiero—y voy a—sanar.

I inherited the need to howl from my grandmother, but instead of drawing blood, I want to—and I will—heal. I will love myself into a garden.

In a garden, any number of things can grow, from blades of grass to vines curling up the trees. If you put your hand in the soil, it can slip between your fingers like dust, or it could be that deep, rich soil que huele a tierra después de la lluvia. There are just as many types of gardens as there are people. What grows in the garden relies on the seeds that are planted, the amount of rain, where the sun shines, the present season, and, most importantly, the soil.

Two seeds buried in the same ground will not grow exactly the same, just as two seeds in different types of soil will turn out completely distinct. Each seed takes the nutrients it needs and turns into a fruit, a flower, or a plant that thrives in the garden it's in. The cactus that grows in the desert wilts in the frost, just like the mango tree can't hold roots in the dry sand. The same works for you. It is important you learn what your seeds need to bloom.

The soil your garden is growing in is your foundation. In it are all the things you have learned, consciously and unconsciously, about yourself and the world around you. These lessons that keep us from finding our voice and changing the way we see ourselves and others stem from internalized oppression. They are the thoughts, ideas, and beliefs that were planted into our soil by culture, family, friends, and society that deplete us of our potential, telling us that we are lesser than because of what we look like, how we act, or who we love. We internalize oppression when we look at ourselves through the eyes of the oppressor that divides us from true self and community. We shrink ourselves to fit the boxes society created and deemed as valuable.

For instance, my immigrant parents believed what the white people said. We grew up trying to be like them. We feared them and felt like they had power over people like us. Our skin needed to be lighter. When we spoke, our accents needed to be undetectable. Our dreams needed to be the same—married, with a picket fence around a perfect house, a dog, and a so-called good job. Our minds still saw them as our colonizers, whom we had to serve. We grew up in constant change, taught to never find joy in who we are, but trying to morph into something we couldn't be. Into something that, deep down, we didn't want to be, representative of our fucked-up history. But that is what power is—the ability to say what matters and what doesn't.

Pero ya no. We define who we are one day at a time.

Unlearning internalized oppression is like digging out the roots of a weed from within ourselves. Much of what we know and understand is so deep because of the simple fact that this was the foundation we were programmed to have for the rest of our lives. Some of us learned the principles that feed our internalized oppression through violence, where acting out in any other way but the expected resulted in a lack of safety or fear. Others learned through examples, like watching the way the mujeres in their lives never strayed from roles that were made for them.

Since these perceptions are a part of how we present ourselves to the world, the process of evaluating them and changing them, or the awareness of how they came to be, is vulnerable work. A lot of times, it's not a linear process, but a constant practice of understanding your current self and the self you want to be as you move through new experiences in life.

There can be a comfort in knowing the role you've been given in life, whether that role makes you happy or not. Taking such a close examination can be scary because sometimes our current way of thinking is so tied to what we consider our core values, or the traits, beliefs, and thoughts that make us unique. There can be a fear that comes with the unknown, a fear of standing up for yourself, a fear of embracing emotions, or of losing parts of yourself and being rejected by loved ones. All of these pieces are valid because they are part of the metamorphosis.

Yet, you deserve to look at yourself and your people con ojos de amor. Eyes of love that see a version of yourself that does not shrink. Eyes of love that see your family, your community, your cultura, your ancestors in a new and informed perspective. Como una persona digna de libertad, igualdad y felicidad. So, let's look closer. Let's get to know the soil you were born into and the environmental conditions that made it what it is. Specifically, the machismo, marianismo, racismo, homophobia, and familismo that whisper in our ears y se encajan en nuestros corazones como espinas sin darnos cuenta.

Entonces, aquí estamos, mujeres que ya se cansaron de seguir sangrando. Mujeres valientes que están listas para sanar. We must tend to our wounds with cariño and without a rush. Eres una flor en su proceso. Primero tenemos que conocer las raíces y las semillas de tu jardín. We must become acquainted with the tierra you were born into. We will see what you inherited and what may need uprooting in order for the flowers to bloom.

MACHISMO

Say this with me: machistas are mugre—machistas are dirt. Very few seeds can grow from dirt. Yet our cultura has tried to grow marriages, families, religion, and countries on machista dirt. Machismo is the belief that men are superior and entitled to hold power over women. Sadly, many of us have been hearing machista shit since we were in our mothers's wombs. We were born into machista dirt and have machismo scars and bleeding wounds. Most of us, if not all of us, also have some roots of internalized machismo. We need to turn that machista shit into fertilizer—only then will our seeds grow.

"Ojalá sea niño. Las niñas son más difíciles. Da miedo traer a una niña a este mundo."

"I hope it is a boy, because it is more dangerous and challenging to bring a girl into this world."

This little statement has deep roots. It is one of the first seeds that is planted, often before we are born, and it embodies a lot of what machismo looks and feels like in many culturas. On the surface, it's not only a preference for a boy, but an acknowledgement that the world we live in today is not a safe place for a girl. The soil does not have what a girl would need to flourish. This statement tells us: *If I bring a girl into this world, I will have to do more work to raise her to be "good" and "protect" her from the men.*

There is an unwavering understanding in Latine culture that having a boy is easier and less work. This is because there are fewer rules and societal pressures when it comes to raising good Latino boys. Boys that later become men are seen as the ones who carry on the family legacy and lead as the head of the household. As such, boys are treated like kings, and girls are expected to serve them.

Machismo is the belief that men are superior and entitled to hold power over women. It is a distinct cultural label that describes how traditions, religion, economic distribution, and family dynamics feed into greater gender discrimination. In Latine communities, it is the blueprint that tells men and women how their values, attitudes, and relationship to masculinity are supposed to operate. Informed by its colonial history, the concept of machismo works within a strict binary that doesn't acknowledge or respect the existence of other genders or queer expression.

A lot of times, machismo appears in the distinctly different ways both genders are raised. Boys are often given a lot of grace as far as their curfews, who they hang with, and the mistakes they make. Mothers may show more outward affection toward their sons by giving them words of encouragement, cooking for them, or taking their side without question during conflicts.

In contrast, a daughter may be ruled by a completely different standard within the same family. Who her friends are, how she dresses, and whether she "talks back" are all determined by the people she lives with. There is an inherent expectation that domestic needs like cooking, cleaning, or taking care of others are her job. These expectations are not consistently communicated within a family unit—the daughter should already know her place, which has been modeled for her by her mamá, her tías, and her abuelas.

Some of the palabras most commonly heard in households are:

"Pobrecito." Poor thing.

"Así son los hombres." That's the way men are.

"Los hombres no lloran." Men don't cry.

"Ese es trabajo de mujer, mijo. Tú no limpias." That's a woman's job, son. You don't clean.

"No es tu culpa; ella se lo merece por fácil." It's not your fault; that woman deserves it because she looks easy.

Machismo teaches us to protect men instead of holding them accountable. Machismo teaches women it is their job to protect and fix broken men. Sometimes we build up these men just so they can break us again and again.

Expressions of machismo may vary from family to family and region to region across Latin America, but the core is the same: As a part of the overarching patriarchy, what a man says, does, and desires is prioritized over what a woman wants, needs, or dreams of.

When the seed of machismo begins to grow, it branches into different areas. Novelas, for example, are a perfect depiction of the hypermasculinity seeping into daily entertainment. Many of the classic novelas we grew up with follow a similar formula: The man is the hero and the story centers on him, his problems, and his journey to solve them, while a cast of women orbit his life, competing with one another to be the chosen one.

Although certain shows have modified this structure, whether it's swapping a hero for a heroine or making the love interest more adventurous, the model of masculinity is still rooted in machismo. It is the kind of toxic masculinity that highlights aggression, dominance, and control. It conflates power with violence and takes skills like listening, sharing, and communicating sadness, fear, or doubt as signs of weakness. The impact of watching this dynamic play out in both real life and in fictional stories can't be understated. Given the popularity of novelas and the ritual of sitting down at a particular day and time to watch the next episode, novelas become a reaffirming tool that paint a picture of what love, family, and gender roles should look like.

Due to its presence in what we listen to, watch, and learn from others, most, if not all of us, have some internalized machismo. Digging up those roots requires a lot of unlearning and cariño, largely because of how intertwined machismo is in our cultura. This is one of the reasons we struggle to untangle ourselves from it. Our cultural and family system is deeply enmeshed with machista beliefs. I pray we work actively to create a world in which anyone can bloom into the flower they were meant to become. Que si un humano viene a este mundo, se sienta suficientemente seguro para ser quien es y tratar a los demás con amor y respeto... y ya. Su género no tiene nada que ver.

The questions then become:

How do I see the world?
How do I see myself?
Am I the person I want to be, or am I the person other people
    want me to be?

The majority of the time, we are not asked about who we are as women or what we'd like. We are told. They tell us who we should be and how we should be. There's a list of qualities dictating what "good" and "bad" women are. Ni nos preguntan; solo nos dicen. At times, it can feel like there is only one way to be a woman. Ideas of femininity can seem quite inflexible and established. It is assumed that by being born women, we are destined to follow the one, well-paved path set out for us. On this path, the rules are pretty clear: Society tells us to dress in pink and to like boys. Our families tell us that we are fragile and that the most important thing is to be beautiful.

It feels like we are not allowed to decide who we are and that we have few options for who we can be. We are often judged or condemned if we deviate from the oppressive cage of femininity and womanhood we are born into. As Latinas, I can almost write a list of rules I was taught growing up, over and over again, about how to be a "good woman," "una buena hija," "una buena esposa," pero nunca nadie me preguntó qué tipo de mujer quería ser. Nobody ever asked me what type of woman I wanted to be. I never asked myself. I simply did what I was told. I aimed to please the people around me as a survival mechanism, another rule for being a good woman. When we subscribe to this lifestyle of being a good woman, we are actually subscribing to toxic femininity.

I say toxic femininity to refer to the concept of adhering to this rigid, gender-binary societal standard of femininity and womanhood. It is a manifestation of internalized machismo. Toxic femininity upholds patriarchal systems and values. No seas una mujer tóxica. You are oppressing yourself and the mujeres around you when you let others tell you what type of woman you should be. This is an invitation to stop trying to be a good woman. Porque en realidad estás convirtiendo a la feminidad en una versión tóxica que pone veneno en el progreso de la liberación colectiva de las mujeres. Toxic femininity is a poison to the liberation of womankind—we want to move away from the binary, not uphold it. Be the type of woman you are. Be the type of woman who is free. Be whoever the fuck you want to be.

Yo quiero un mundo donde las mujeres puedan ser y hacer lo que les dé su chingada gana. I want a world where women can be and do whatever they fuck they want. Where your dreams, your hopes, your thoughts, your words matter. You matter; the past you, the current you, and the version of you that you're building through this work.

Machismo raises women that act as windbreakers for fragile men, protecting them while sacrificing ourselves. Mujeres are taught to silence and shrink ourselves for the sake of serving the male ego. Qué triste. You are so much more than submissive calladitas.

I grew up seeing the women in my family sacrifice themselves over and over again. Their voices, dreams, wants, and needs weren't as important as the men they had to serve and protect. In machista mugre, the only thing that grows is the male ego, while women's dreams wither. Los sueños de una mujer no pueden sobrevivir cuando son plantados en una tierra machista.

Far too often, a strong woman who is actively resisting and challenging machismo is seen as a threat which must be tamed. A mujer who is actively anti-machista is a wildfire threatening a whole ecosystem of dry, shallow plants. She is a mujerista. Ready to catch fire and burn to the ground. Liberty is contagious. Liberty is a direct threat to oppressors. A mujer who is badass and beautiful y lo sabe makes machistas tremble. This woman is the flower de las semillas nuevas que estamos plantando.

When we get to this place, we have begun planting new seeds. We need to turn that machista shit into fertilizer—only then will our garden continue to grow.

MARIANISMO

I have a tía, and I'm sure you have a tía like her too, who is the ideal woman. The most loving, generous, hardworking, nurturing, and humble individual. Para lo que necesiten, ella allí está.

Every morning, she rises before the sun. When my great-grandmother was alive, my tía, by herself, would cook three meals a day, bathe her, and take her to her appointments. During the week, she would teach kindergarten, paying special attention to each student and their families. After work, she would pick up her grandchildren and watch them until their parents got home, cooking dinner for each person and a little extra for them to take back. Once they were all back in their respective homes, she would stay up past midnight planchando la ropa.

I know all this because I spent a whole day with her once. I was exhausted from just watching her. Exhausted and deeply concerned.

This was especially true when I saw her ironing her husband's underwear.

¡No puede ser! I screamed in my mind.

"Tía, ¿eres feliz?" I asked her one day.

"Ay, mija, la felicidad no tiene nada que ver. Esta es mi vida."

She didn't even look up. She had come to accept that she didn't deserve her own happiness.

I grew up seeing the women in my family sacrifice themselves over and over again. Their voice, dreams, wants, and needs weren't as important as the men they had to serve and protect. When they received praise, it was because they had followed the rules, or did tasks without being asked.

If machismo is the rule book for masculinity, then marianismo is the bible for femininity. Under marianismo, virtue and purity are the core ideals that women are expected to uphold through their words, thoughts, and actions. The term comes from La Virgen María, or the story of the Virgin Mary, who gave birth to Jesus. Her lack of sex is the key part of her divinity and qualifies her to be the mother of Christ. A staple figure in Catholicism, La Virgen María paints the ultimate picture of purity, abstinence, and submission. She obediently follows her holy destiny and paves the way for a male savior.

From the leadership of their fathers to the successive leadership of their husbands, women learn to seek approval and permission from male figures from a very young age. Following the guiding principles of marianismo, a woman waits until she is married to have sex, because sex is an indication of moral stature, and it needs to be saved for the husband. Once married, the ideal woman is submissive to her husband and devotes her time and attention to his needs. In this space, the ideal woman is judged based on how selfless she is, her chastity, her appearance as a desirable but virtuous woman, and her ability to cater to other people.

The more calladita she is, the more beautiful she seems. The woman is praised for being so selfless and for all that she does for everyone else. If this woman takes time to rest, pursue her interests, or express her opinion, she is demonized and cut down, either verbally, physically, or both by members of her family and community. Quietness gives the surrounding people the opportunity to shape the ideal woman into something of their choosing. A blank slate.

I like to call this transformation the "señora effect." It's as if, when you get married or get to a certain age, there is a societal shift and expectation that you become "a woman" and you are expected to look, dress, and be a certain way. There are strict spoken and unspoken rules. In my case, one day I was a recent college graduate. The next day, I was a señora with my mom and grandmother pressuring me to make my husband food, talking to me about the best ways to take stains out of clothes, and the worst part: ¡¿Por qué no le planchas su ropa?! Suddenly, they weren't concerned that I had just graduated from an Ivy League university. They only talked to me about cooking, cleaning, and serving my husband.

All other women that do not fit this saint archetype fall into the category of the puta, the bitch, the slut, the woman with no morals y ya. A social outcast. There are no options. To be seen as anything other, to be as equally important a human being as men, and not just a source of endless energy and support for her family and her husband's needs, is to be the enemy. To speak up is to be the enemy.

The convenience of marianismo is that it hands women their identity in a neat list of Dos and Don'ts. As feminist activist Betty Friedan wrote in *The Feminine Mystique*, "even the very admission of women's intelligence and individuality is a problem."[1] Individuality can feel unattainable when what is right and what is wrong has been drilled into a woman's mind for so long. The comfort of knowing that, if certain goal posts are met, goodness can be achieved, can make marianismo a tempting reason to never question its existence nor consider resistance. If the basis of it is centered on being good, why would we want to do any differently?

Con razón, Latinas are at higher risk for mental health struggles such as depression and anxiety.[2] We are under chronic psychological distress due to the pressure to self-silence and self-sacrifice in order to be respected and accepted. We are taught to aguantar domestic violence, sexual violence, and emotional abuse instead of standing up for ourselves. It's hard not to be depressed when you are told your main purpose in life is to serve men and be quiet.

The fruits of marianismo are not necessarily the problem. The roots or the fact that it is a seed planted within us are the real problem. Cooking, cleaning, and taking care of others can be a source of joy. These actions may be part of the way a woman expresses love, appreciation, and respect. The problem comes from marianismo's attempt to use the idea of goodness and virtue to force women to do things without ever straying from the prescribed track.

Over the years, my mother and grandmother have witnessed my healing journey. Initially, they resisted because most of my self-love choices are different and contrary to what they were told was right. They couldn't understand why I would willingly make things harder for myself instead of just being "happy and grateful."

No entendían por qué quería pensar en mis heridas o tomarlas en cuenta. Para sanar. Ellas me preguntaban: "Pero ¿por qué?" Porque me amo. Y ya me cansé de vernos sangrar. Nuestras mamis cargan las heridas de sus mamis … y nosotras también.

Cuando nosotras sanamos, ellas también. Healing ourselves can lead the women around us to consider doing the same for themselves.

RACISM

Racism and colorism have deep and influential roots that take hold in our culture. The preference for proximity to whiteness can be found in entertainment, the arts, politics, and in our families. Within our homes, there can be a preference for family members that have lighter skin tones, an admiration for people with ojos de color, or declarations that los blanquitos son más bonitos. No son más bonitos. Son más privilegiados. However, most of us grew up believing this was true. Many of us were raised to believe white was right and better and beautiful—and we were not. This is, in short, internalized racism.

The Racial and Cultural Identity Development Theory developed by Dr. William Cross Jr.[3] identifies some key stages people of color walk through as they become aware of and cultivate their own sense of identity. It is not a one-size-fits-all formula, but it does provide a useful framework from which to build upon. These key stages are:

1. **Pre-encounter:** This is the stage in which you don't think much about race or the racial implications for your existence. There is a general conformity with the white dominant culture. This is the stage in which internalized oppression blinds us and has us believing "white is right" and that there is something wrong with anything and anyone who does not fit the dominant standards. During

this stage many people of color are too preoccupied with trying to be, sound, look, and act white that they do not embrace or foster connection to their own culture. On the contrary, we distance ourselves and water down whatever makes us different.

Perhaps you are still in this stage. Perhaps it happened early in your life. It is a privilege to not have to think of race. In some ways, it is also a desired destination. We need to imagine a world in which matters of racial identity didn't consume us with fear, violence, and oppression. In a way, the pre-encounter is a privileged and childlike view of the world. There is an innocence about not being preoccupied by your race or your neighbor's skin color.

2. **Encounter:** At some point, the innocence gets shattered. We realize that race is still very much a life-or-death matter for many. Race colors how we view the world and ourselves. The encounter can come as a shock to your system. There is grief in realizing the color of your skin and cultural background make you visible and invisible at the same time. This grief can double when you realize there is conflict inside of your own culture, especially for women that identify as Afro-Latinas. In *Sister Outsider: Essays and Speeches*, Audre Lorde writes, "Within this country where racial difference creates a constant, if unspoken, distortion of vision, Black women have on one hand always been highly visible, and so, on the other hand, have been rendered invisible through the depersonalization of racism."[4] Afro-Latinas have to balance the racial intricacies and prejudices of being Black in a white-dominated

society with the colorism that can occur within their very own families. The encounter experience can occur as a reaction to an outside event or to something from within our homes by the very people we were taught to trust: our families.

3. **Immersion/Emersion**: The immersion stage of your identity development consists of you actively seeking to learn about your cultura and how you relate to it on a personal level. How does your culture influence who you are? The immersion stage involves curiosity and exploration. During this stage, you may lean in a little closer, look a little deeper into your cultural roots, and listen more attentively when your abuela shares her stories about cuando ella era niña, her novelas, her tierra o le subes el volumen a sus canciones de limpieza de los sábados por la mañana. There may be a desire to speak your mother's native tongue, en mi caso un poquito más de español, o Spanglish. Perhaps you didn't grow up feeling super connected to your culture and a triggering incident happened which prompted you to acercarte un poquito más que antes. The immersion stage is brought on by an encounter which acts as a catalyst for the self-exploration and confrontation of our racial and ethnic identity development. These encounters can invite people to lean in and learn more about their cultura. They can also frighten people into rejecting their cultural connection and further assimilate into the dominant culture. This is often a survival strategy. There are people in environments or situations in which deviating too far from the dominant culture can put them in physical and/or social danger.

4. **Internalization-Commitment**: This is when we have developed a secure sense of our racial and ethnic identity and are comfortable internalizing it and externalizing it. We can navigate diverse social settings within and outside our racial group without having our sense of identity disrupted or threatened. During this stage, the individual feels secure in their sense of ethnic identity, which also becomes an important component of their self-identity. There is a sense of stability, an inner knowing, and the capacity to communicate effectively who you are and what you need. Once you reach this stage in your identity development, you can confidently share what your ethnic and cultural connections are and how you embody them in your life and your being.

Internalization and commitment can feel like creating a space within yourself to house your cultura. It is an embrace rather than resistance. No matter where you are in the world or within yourself, you know who you are and your cultura lives within you. You no longer hide it or experience shame when your ethnicity or culture is brought up o cuando sobresale como fuera de lo normal. There is a congruence that feels like internal peace. There is also a commitment to continue to deepen and expand this connection to your culture within yourself. Integrating your culture with your identity, self, environment, and worldview provides a sense of wholeness and fulfillment to most. It is almost impossible to exclude your culture from your identity.

Not everyone goes through all these stages, nor does each stage look the same for everyone. However, we will use them as a general guide. There is a big possibility you already began your racial and cultural identity development and didn't even know it. The color of our skin, the accent on our words, and the culture we are born into influence the way we take up space in this world and the way this world allows us to take up space. You are blessed with your culture, tu bandera, tu identidad, the melanin on your skin, the thickness of your accent, your thighs, and your hair, and you bless the world each time you decide to take up space. Our cultures directly or indirectly also give us information on who we are, how we should be, and what our roles in our families and relationships should be. The following example is my personal experience with the five stages.

I was in my pre-encounter stage up until middle school. Growing up in the San Fernando Valley, North Hollywood, and Pacoima specifically, my classrooms and surrounding community were primarily Latine. Over 10 percent of San Fernando Valley families lived well below the poverty level, making less than $15,000 a year.[5] My family (and most of my friends' families) were part of that 10 percent. When we started elementary school, our moms would pin our reduced lunch tickets onto our uniform shirts so we wouldn't lose them.

A lot of our families depended on those reduced lunches to survive. After school, the lucky ones who got a dollar would run to los paleteros and buy Hot Cheetos con limón, elotes, paletas, o churros. We would compete to see whose fingers turned reddest from the Hot Cheeto dust and excitedly lick our crusty fingers. Our moms waited for us outside, chismeando in Spanish while we finished our after-school chucherías.

We all understood each other. All of my teachers spoke some level of Spanish. There was a sense of unity. No one really felt "othered" based on their race. I barely had to think about race. This was my childlike memory of that season of life: coexistence.

My encounter occurred during PE in sixth grade. Walter Reed Middle School offered a program for its highly gifted students. I begged my mom to let me enroll because the smartest kids in my school were going there and I wanted to be one of them.

The joke was on me because I was the only Latina in the classroom. This was a first for me. I had never seen kids so white. They looked, talked, and dressed like the kids from my favorite shows on TV. They wore clothes from stores I was too scared to even try to pronounce, like Abercrombie. Many of their parents worked in Hollywood, had nice cars, and talked like the TV parents, showing up at school conferences and student concerts looking fabulous. In comparison, my family was big and loud, and my parents came to the same events with their dirty, greasy work clothes. My mom had a thick accent and always looked lost. None of my teachers spoke Spanish. I learned to translate. I also learned shame and felt embarrassed by my family and how different we were from everyone else.

The shame was cemented one day during PE. My best friends and I were running our daily laps. One of them was Korean and the other Italian. When they saw some Latino boys messing around, they rolled their eyes, turned to me, and said, "At least you're not like those Mexicans. You know what they say about Mexicans."

I felt as if someone had just dumped iced water on me. Shocked.

The encounter.

What did they say?

Who were they?

Why were they talking about us?

I was afraid to hear the answer, but I had to know.

"What do they say about Mexicans?" I asked apprehensively.

They proceeded to list off stereotype after stereotype:

Lazy.

Poor.

Violent.

Cholos.

Not as smart.

Loud.

Angry.

Dangerous.

Drug addicts and alcoholics.

Trouble.

Illegal.

At that point, I didn't know they were stereotypes. They said them with such certainty, I thought they were truths. The venom of internalized oppression had entered my system. My heart sank and panicked. I knew that it wasn't true or fair. Not all of us are like that.

But I also knew some of that could be true. My family was poor, loud, and sometimes violent. My neighbors were cholos. There was an internal battle going on inside me as I kept running laps beside these friends that all of a sudden didn't feel so friendly.

I wanted to run away and cry.

I also wanted to be far, far away from those stereotypes.

I wanted to prove I was a good Mexican.

They didn't have to be afraid of me or look down on me. From then on, I was no longer proud of my red Hot Cheeto fingers. After school, I washed my hands really well so they wouldn't notice them the next day. Deep down, I felt heartbroken. Some of those things did apply to me, my friends, my family. However, it felt so wrong because they didn't know us. We were people trying to survive battles they would never understand. We were doing our best. My cholo neighbors were actually very nice to me. One of them would even write to me from jail. Our other neighbor's baby drowned in her bathtub. The mother came to our apartment screaming hysterically. My mom held her as she sobbed while the ambulance took her baby girl away. We watched her twin toddler boys for a few days. Our other neighbor's husband would hit her. She would send her kids to our house when things got too dangerous at her home. We helped her eldest boy with his homework, since she didn't speak any English. Every now and then she would thank us with homemade tamales. These were my people. This was my community.

We are humans with stories, pain, wounds, dreams, kind eyes, secrets, battles, and so much more than meets the eye. All these thoughts, stories, memories, and humans ran through my mind as I ran on the field. I felt the weight of racism on my shoulders. It was heavy. It made it harder to keep going. This encounter marked the day I began trying to prove myself worthy. It opened my eyes to the vast grip that race, class, and privilege had on everyone. It was everywhere. I couldn't unsee it now.

My mom worked at Valley Foods as a cashier, at Winchell's Donuts, and as a secretary for abusive bosses who would constantly threaten to call the migra on her. She would come home crying and feeling like shit. We were scared one of these days the migra would come. There was even a plan in place if that happened: go to the neighbor's house and hide until they leave, then call mi Tita. Thankfully, they never came.

These fears, threats, and constant degradation taught us to shrink and get out of the way. We never wanted to make a white person mad at us because they had the power to ruin our lives. Somehow, we had all accepted this was how things were supposed to be. This acceptance of being constantly oppressed is a learned helplessness resulting from internalized oppression. Believing we deserve to be treated as if we were less than and being a target of racism has deep detrimental effects on an individual's and community' self-perception and mental wellness.

Race is a social construct without biological meaning. Take a minute to reflect on the moment of your first encounter y abrázate. This is a crucial time in your development. Your initial encounter with systemic racism can often lead to internalized oppression influencing your sense of identity like a deadly venom or cancerous weed. You may have repeated racist things about others or even to yourself in an attempt to fit in. You may have tried to look, be, or sound more "right." You may have tried to distance yourself from being too different. Perhaps you still do. Uproot what needs uprooting and replace it with the truth you know now. Abrázate y forgive yourself for all the shame and the seeds of self-hate that you planted. This is a beautiful time to explore those seeds. It is a time to grieve how things could have been if someone had taught us to love our skin and wrap our cultura around us con orgullo, como un rebozo. You are allowed to grieve the years you lost trying to be someone you are not instead of loving the beautiful person you've always been.

There is rage from being born into a world which didn't accept you and made you believe there was something wrong with you. There is rage in the knowledge that racism continues and that there are still BIPOC children who believe they are less worthy than their white peers. There is rage and shame and grief in the tears watering this garden.

There is also hope. There is hope in the awareness that you hold, right here, right now. There is hope because you are becoming a woman who loves herself—you are becoming a revolution. Es un proceso, un desarrollo. You are a work in progress. We all are. Our cultura identity development is a nonlinear process of becoming, unbecoming, unlearning, unraveling, and relearning who the fuck we are.

HOMOPHOBIA

Many of us queer seres were not given language or tools to develop our queer identity growing up. The language we were given was often homophobic, derogatory, or shameful. The tools were mostly weapons meant to change us and harm us. It is hard to accept and love yourself fully when you grow up hearing there is something wrong with you. Being queer in a Latine household can be heartbreaking.

Queer theory, first coined by Teresa de Lauretis[6], aims to deconstruct what is socially acceptable as "normal" when it comes to concepts such as heterosexuality, homosexuality, gender, and sexuality. It also aims to reconstruct new ways of thinking, defining, and reclaiming these concepts essential to identity development and identity politics. Queer theory moves us away from the binary and challenges the heteronormative power structures in place. Gracia Trujillo, profesora de sociología de la Universidad Complutense de Madrid y activista feminista queer, defines "queer" as "…esa rareza, esa desviación de la normalidad, de lo straight, en términos sexuales y genéricos."[7] She goes on to define homophobia as an arbitrary man-ifestation that consists of signaling the other as contrary, inferior, or abnormal.[8]

Parte de la magia de ser queer es que parte de su definición es no ser "normal," while at the same time we normalize our queerness. Trujillo writes about how one of the least queer things to do is to try to define queer and put us in a box.[9] Queerness is weirdness, deviation from the societal structures in place. It is meant to stay outside of boxes, bina-ries, and definitions. It is simply meant to exist. Trujillo takes it fur-ther and claims queer is better used as a verb: queering. To be queer. To exist in a state of queerness. I am queering right now. If you are queer, you too are queering. We are queering together. Qué bonito.

Trujillo's "anti-definition" of queerness is as follows: "Queer is a political position and an epistemology (a tool, or toolkit, which may help us observe and interpret the world in a different form, in a critical form). It is a process, an acción, not an identity. And a verb, to queer, or 'queering' which means to transcend, question, contaminate...tortillear o mariconear."[10]

Nonbinary beings queer beautifully. They live outside the binary boxes. I believe nonbinary beings are the closest humans get to God because they create who they are and move with fluidity: pueden ser todo y nada a la vez. They decide on she/he/they/them. Being nonbinary es badass y bonito. Elles mismes escogen vivir fuera de las cajas binarias en las que fueron colocades desde que nacieron: niña, niño, azul, rosita, etc. Elles son les valientes que se atrevieron a transcender y existir en esos espacios liminales de sexo, género e identidad. They are the brave ones who dared to transcend and exist in the liminal spaces of sex, gender, and identity. This is quintessen-tial queer shit.

Trujillo encourages us to see queerness as a change of perspective away from "normal" individuals and sexual minorities to a more collective view on accepting everyone as they are.[11] Once we accept that every single person is different and nobody is truly normal, or abnormal, then we will be able to see society as a whole, rather than point out individuals. In a heteropatriarchal, classist, and racist system, we must be willing to question and deconstruct these values and how they inform our sense of self. Heteronormativity, according to American literary critic Michael Warner, consists of "all the processes which normalize and maintain heterosexuality as an elemental form for humanity, it is seen as the model for human relationships between genders, it is the invisible base upon which society is built and the only means of reproduction which without society wouldn't exist."[12] Being queer is not fitting into this societal norm. Most of us do not want to fit in.

However, there is such a thing as "homonormativity," according to Lisa Duggan, Professor of Social and Cultural Analysis at New York University. This term refers to queers who, instead of wanting to deconstruct heteronormativity, simply adopt and uphold it.[13] They do not wish to dismantle the system, but rather fit into it and be good little gays. They want that invitation to the hetero party. Sometimes this is an externalization of survival mechanisms, internalized homophobia, or simply a safer way of queering. There are gays who accept their homosexuality, yet they hate that they are gay. I've heard queer men and women say, "I hate being gay. I know that I am, so I have to accept it and live with it, but I really want the hetero lifestyle." One of my friends confessed he wanted to marry a woman and have kids and have that cookie-cutter life. He would still like to fuck men and sleep around, but with a wife and kids on the side. When you choose to unsubscribe from the heteronormative life, you choose to put yourself at risk for discrimination and may lose privileges and rights. You choose to unlearn most of what you were taught about who you are, who you should be, what is right, wrong, acceptable, love, sex, marriage, beautiful, etc. Entering your queerness is an act of love, deconstruction, and revolution. It is a whole new world.

Despite the prevalence of queer influence and impact on culture, from drag queens on daytime television to the flamboyance of Walter Mercado, actual queer Latines and their experiences with homophobia are intertwined with familismo, machismo, and religion.

Familismo is a cultural belief that holds loyalty to the family system above all. Family spends time with family, family supports family, and most importantly, what happens within the family stays within the family. The strength of one particular family is based on how close each member is to one another and what they are willing to do for one another. A lot of times, your loyalty feels like the greatest honor you can give your family. Having a queer person in your family—which can be seen as a direct opponent to the masculinity of machismo, religious teachings, or necessity for a man, depending on the queer expression—is a threat to that structure, since it goes against the greater cultural expectation and potentially attracts shame from the surrounding community.

Shame for being perceived as a family threat or burden is one of the biggest reasons many Latines remain closeted or come out of the closet late in life. Some families treat having a queer person in the family as if it was something bad, yet they will go out of their way to protect the abusers, pedophiles, and violent people within the family system. All in the name of family, all in the name of "love." Due to traumatic encounters with shame, many queer folks internalize homophobia and baptize themselves with shame. Many times, we believe there is something wrong and unnatural about us simply because we are queer. I've crossed paths with many queer folks who are homophobic, just like I've met many queer folks who began hating themselves as a result of their experiences at church. It breaks my heart because I know it is not their fault. When you only hear negative things, like "asco," "shame," and "ungodly," it is difficult not to start believing them. There is a deep cognitive dissonance when your identity, who you love, and your community seem to go against one another.

Because of its perceived danger to the family, queerness is not presented as a viable option for many of us. It is too disruptive. This is reaffirmed by strict religious instruction, which tells us not to hate, yet teaches us to only love those who fit into very specific boxes. Paired with the idea of disobeying familismo, many family members utilize religion to compound the shame, trying to frame queerness as a betrayal of both family and God, as a moral failing that can be prayed away. Since I refused to pray my gay away, both of my parents took the job of "saving" me very seriously and had Bible study groups praying for my salvation. I felt ashamed to like girls and I felt ashamed to have a mother who hated girls who liked girls.

"How can you say such cruel things when the Bible teaches us to love our neighbors? Jesus didn't make an exception for who our neighbors are. How can you say you love God when you say such hateful things about his children?" I asked my mami one day.

She simply said, "I'm not perfect. I like the gay guys, pero las lesbianas nunca me han gustado."

Oftentimes, there is a unique kind of homophobia when it comes to queer women. Las pinches lesbianas. Some theories believe this is the case because it is the only identity that does not want or require a man—in fact, we reject them. The concept of a woman existing without a man, let alone loving another woman, is in direct contrast to what machismo and marianismo demand. Many lesbian women grow up hearing words like machorra, marimacha, maricona. These words plant seeds of hate and fear within ourselves. When you grow up hearing who you are is bad, sinful, or disrespectful, it is nearly impossible to love and feel proud of yourself. Some of us grow up hating our queerness or hating ourselves for being queer. The homophobes in our lives make us feel like this is the right thing to do. There is no pride, just shame. There is a desire to change or a sense of failure for not being straight. "Me gustan las mujeres, pero no quiero ser lesbiana." The word lesbian more often than not was said in a whisper, as if it was a bad word. They said lesbian the same way my mother did: con asco. It felt dirty. It was uttered like a curse. I don't think I grew up hearing one positive thing about lesbians or queer women. It wasn't until I started saying them to myself. Yo empecé a decir cosas bonitas de mí por ser lesbiana. This is how I broke the curse. I began planting new seeds.

It took me years to accept myself as a queer woman. It took years of therapy and intentional self-awareness to realize I like women. I love women. I want to be with women. ¡Ay, Dios mío! Soy lesbiana. Gracias a Dios, soy lesbiana. Soy una pinche lesbiana, ¿y qué?

When that moment of acceptance finally arrived, it felt like I was too late. I was a nice Christian woman married to a nice Christian man. Nice Christian women do not fantasize about being with other women instead of their husbands. I felt so much shame. Shame is a manifestation of internalized oppression. Shame tells us we are unlovable. It tells us to hide our true selves and become a more palatable version of ourselves. So I did.

We have to actively love ourselves as queer women in order to undo the damage done by internalized homophobia. Nobody in my family was going to celebrate my queerness. So, I did. Nobody was going to tell me beautiful things about being a pinche lesbiana. Más bien, it always came with warnings and threats. It felt like it was the worst thing I could be and like I was actively attacking my family by being queer. Tal vez it was the same for you. We have to be the ones to tell ourselves cosas bonitas about our queerness. Llena ese corazoncito queer con semillas de amor.

Mujer, in case you haven't heard cosas bonitas about being a lesbian o mujer queer, and in case you don't know where to start, I wrote this for us:

> Dear queer inner niña,
>> Pienso en ti, y solo quiero abrazarte y llenarte de besitos.
>> On your cheeks y en las orillas de tus ojos, por donde caen
>>> tus lágrimas,
>> esas lágrimas que piensas que nadie ve.
>> Pienso en ti y quiero recordarte que tienes alas.
>> I want to remind you that you have wings and maybe
>>> right now
>> you feel like you are ese gusanillo feo that may never turn
>>> into a
>> mariposa.
>> I remember feeling like I was that gusanito that was never
>>> going to
>> fly, or the one that was never going to come out of the
>>> cocoon.
>> Pero, I promise, you do get your wings.
>> And you will learn how to fly.
>> I have spent my whole life fighting for your wings.
>> I want to take off the burdens you've been carrying.
>> They were never meant for you to carry.

As the firstborn and eldest daughter,
    you had to be responsible for too much too soon.
Casi no tuviste tiempo de ser una niña.
Y mucho menos de ser una niña queer.
Discover who you are: qué te gusta y quién te gusta.
You were so busy taking care of everyone else you didn't learn how
to take care of yourself.
You were busy being what everyone else told you you should be.
There is nothing wrong with you for choosing who you love.
I'm sorry I let the fear instilled by religion and cultura keep my
identity from blooming.
I hid behind the color pink, boys, and everything I thought would
keep me in the closet.
Your queerness doesn't make you any less worthy of receiving love.
De ese amor bonito, amor del bueno.
No tengas miedo when you realize you like girls!
Es algo hermoso de ti.
Es algo que no tienes que esconder.
Es algo que también te va a dar alas.
Es hora de abrir esas alas y dejarte amar, y brillar.
Porque este mundo needs more queer girls like you.

During another one of our cafecito times, mi Tita looked at me and told me, "Tu tía Maricela empezó a hablar de ti. Dijo que eras una pinche lesbiana. Si oigo que te vuelve a decir así, le voy a partir su madre." My initial response was to thank her for standing up for me. I stopped and processed. She got mad that mi tía said I was a lesbian. She didn't lie. Her intention and tone were derogatory, but in reality, she was saying the truth.

"Pero ¿por qué te enojas, si soy una pinche lesbiana?"

"Sí, pero no quiero que ande hablando mal de ti."

"Yo no lo tomo a mal porque sí soy una pinche lesbiana. Amo ser quien soy y poder amar a quien me dé la chingada gana."

"Sí, qué bueno, pero de todos modos le voy a partir su madre."

I tried. What I gained from this conversation was an opportunity to name myself and declare a love for my identity as a queer mujer. My grandmother got to see a pinche lesbiana who loves herself. I am a pinche lesbiana who loves herself. Su veneno and shame did not belong to me anymore. I had replaced it with medicine and self-love. Pinche lesbiana became something that brought healing rather than poison. Nos sanamos cuando nos nombramos y reclamamos con amor y orgullo quienes somos.

I had always been told who to be and who not to be. Lesbiana was high on the list of things not to be. Nobody prepared me for the power and agency I felt when I was finally able to name and identify myself as queer or lesbiana out loud to the most important people in my life. Terrifying, claro. Liberating, ¡a huevo! It felt like this was a part of me that was missing and that I had to unearth and somewhat fight for.

I had to fight religious oppression, heteronormativity, and my very own internalized homophobia. This was the undeniable piece of me that I had spent most of my life denying. I denied it because I was afraid. I was afraid because I knew I wouldn't be accepted for who I truly was/am. I was afraid of being rejected and not being loved and disappointing my mom, God, the church, my siblings, my husband, everyone. I was the eldest sister who had to set a good example. So, I denied and repressed. I put on a smile and tried to be the best at everything, for everyone. Until I couldn't anymore. It felt like taking off layers of oppression poco a poquito. Leaving my home. Going to therapy. Getting a divorce. Coming out to myself. Falling in love with a woman. Coming out to my family. Claiming and naming myself and my sexual identity. It felt like a conscious choice to see myself for the first time and intentionally choosing to love myself con todos mis colores y sombras.

For me it felt like a revolution and liberation. For my mother and family, it felt like a desmadre. I went from being the golden child in my family, the firstborn daughter on a pedestal, to the divorcée who was also a pinche lesbiana. When I unsubscribed from the hetero life, I realized how privileged I had been as a nice Christian wife married to a white man. Not only did we benefit from his whiteness, but we also benefitted from being hetero and Christian. We had access to so many resources. My family treated us like we were royalty. They treated my marriage like my biggest accomplishment, more so than graduating from an Ivy League college, or making a bestsellers list. When I left this life, not only did I lose societal privileges, but I also lost privileges within my family system. They used to look at me with pride and admiration. They now look at me with disdain and disapproval—like I had it all and I fucked it up for all of us. Although this is their view on my life from a heteronormative lens, I see things completely differently. When I look at myself in the mirror, I look at myself with pride and peace. I finally see all of me reflected back at me, not bits and pieces. I know and love who I am: queer and queering in every way, more and more every day.

Part of getting to know ourselves involves queering. Entering into it with curiosity and intention. To queer also means to be an ally and advocate, to dismantle existing systems of oppression, and to question the hetero-patriarchal norms from which you may be benefitting. Queer theory is necessary from a political standpoint because queer people and their bodies are still being targeted, murdered, bullied, and tormented simply for existing. We need queer theory to create systems that protect and uplift sex workers, trans rights, alternative families, nonmonogamous relationships, intersex beings, and all the queer beings in the world who are simply trying to be, to love and be loved, and to find safe people and places in this world. We need to be those safe people and create those safe places for ourselves and those around us.

When we connect with ourselves as queer beings, we are able to connect with other queer beings. This is why we often find our chosen family—a collection of beings, often queer, who will see us with eyes of love, hold us when the world rejects us, and become a family system of people who choose to love one another and show up for one another as a family would. They will stand with you and against all the things which hurt and oppress you. Usually, our chosen families are the ones that fight for us when we are too tired to fight for ourselves. They see and know you and love you completely. Audre Lorde, a Black, lesbian, feminist writer describes her chosen family as, "The women who sustained me through that period were Black and white, old and young, lesbian, bisexual, and heterosexual, and we all shared a war against the tyrannies of silence."[14] People who will sustain you and join you as you fight your battles against the tyrannies created to oppress you. We are fighting for our collective liberation because we love ourselves and one another so strongly. I may have lost the approval of my family and church community, but I gained the unconditional love and acceptance of my queer family—and myself.

It is time for you to queer. It doesn't mean you have to be queer, but simply dare to see yourself and the world differently and accept that we are all different. It does not mean more or less normal or abnormal. It simply means to be exactly all of who you are. And if you look in the mirror and find a queer being looking back at you, I hope you look at them with love.

Take a moment to ask yourself the following questions and say the answers out loud or write them down in a notebook or journal:

How am I queer and/or queering?

My cultura is a part of my identity in these ways . . .

What type of mujer am I?

How do I feel about my femininity?

What are the ways I currently connect with my femininity?

When I look in the mirror, I see . . .

Afirmaciones

My tears will water the seeds in the gardens of those who come after me. Together, we will watch our gardens bloom.

> *Mis lágrimas nutrirán las semillas en los jardines de la próxima generación. Juntos veremos nuestros jardines florecer.*

I will listen to myself and trust the voice of my soul.

> *Me escucharé y confiaré en el sonido de la voz de mi alma.*

I will stop asking for permission and live my life for myself, as I please.

> *Dejaré de pedir permiso para vivir mi vida. Viviré como me dé la gana, porque esta vida es mía.*

Chapter 2

Sistemas & Semillas

Look at your abuela's hands—they tell you stories of strength, prayers, tortillas, and of all the times she's held on for dear life. Your mother's hands tell stories of grief, nurturing, lessons, lágrimas, and bendiciones. Your hands look like theirs, yet they tell their own stories. I like to imagine the wrinkles on my abuela's hands as the roots of our family tree and the roadmap to my mother's story and my own. The spots and lunares on her hands form constellations illustrating the places she's been, the people she's known, and the experiences she's lived. It is important to understand these stories. Through these stories, we learn of the wounds, wars, and bendiciones we've inherited.

My grandmother grew up on tough love. Boronitas de amor. Her family was poverty stricken. So much so that her mom would hide fruit from her own children en su cajón de calzones. She grew to be so resentful that she began competing with her children for food and resources. The scarcity mentality became a scarcity lifestyle which influenced how they lived and, most importantly, how they loved. They lived as if there was never enough love, like love, too, was a resource that had to be rationed, hidden, hoarded, and fought for. Somehow, my grandmother survived on crumbs of love. Always hungry for more. My grandmother's heart was severely malnourished. She grew up searching for love and only found lovers who gave her crumbs. She took what she could get and stuck with what she knew. When she brought her own daughter into this world, she gave her boronitas de amor. It is all she knew and all she had.

It is important for us to understand the family systems we are born into. Each system has its way of functioning and dysfunctioning. It is important you become familiar with your familia.

Some of us have families that are nurturing and conducive to growth, who celebrate when we bloom, and allow us to have the space to become the kind of person we'd like to be. Some of us have families that are difficult, harsh, or abusive, who made growing up an act of survival, forcing us to adapt to conditions we did not ask for. Many of us grew up in a setting that may have had both: a mixture of people who upheld and tore us down, or times when living with our families was complicated and contradictory. As a child, you look to your family for love, guidance, and validation. The way that love, guidance, and validation are expressed, or the absence of it, shapes our perspective of ourselves and the people around us, and our ability to welcome new experiences. In order to understand what we value, what we believe, and who we'd like to become, it's important to understand how our families operate, so we can see the parts of ourselves that still need healing.

Each family system is influenced by the most dominant culture it's a part of. In individualistic cultures, children are raised to face outward, prioritize themselves, and create an independent life. From a young age, children in these family systems are taught to find the qualities that make them stand out from larger groups, be self-sufficient and self-reliant, and emphasize personal success, goals, and milestones.

The opposite of individualistic systems are centripetal systems. In a centripetal family system, the expectation is that people will build interdependent lives in which they remain connected and centered around core family values and functions. People raised in these systems are taught to consider how their actions, dreams, and reputations affect the strength of their families. Growing up, there is an awareness of our responsibility for taking care of others, working as a collective unit, and understanding the role a person plays in maintaining the stability and day-to-day functions of the family. Praise and validation are given for accomplishments that give back and uplift the family, whereas punishment, shame, and rejection usually result from acts that hurt a part of the family. Both systems can cultivate helpful and harmful qualities in the people raised within them. People in individualistic systems can struggle to ask for help or experience loneliness, while people in family-centric systems may have trouble achieving their dreams or making decisions without outside input.

Our cultura is especially connected to the value of familismo, which is often considered a family-centric system. Traditional Latine families subscribe to the collectivistic value system, which is family-centered and family first. Children are raised to do things for and with the family more than for themselves, girls especially.

A visualization which works for me is envisioning my family system as a forest: a collection of family trees. The trees closest to you represent your immediate family, while those that are further into the forest are your extended family. Imagine the texture of each trunk, the winding roots, the branches twisting upward, the texture of the leaves and the colors changing as the seasons pass. Maybe some of the roots are intertwined, or the branches have been cut off, or a disease is covering the base, preventing any more growth. Some of the plagues ailing the trees in our forest involve intergenerational trauma. This can spread between generations, between family trees, and between root systems.

Whether you remain a part of your family forest or not, you play a role in your family's functioning and they play a role in yours. You are connected. What happened to them in their pasts helped to shape their present, and what has happened to you will help shape future generations. Rather than excuse the wrong things our families have done to us, taking the time and perspective to understand what trauma and lessons they carry within them allows us to see how trauma continues to live within us.

Engaging in the healing process is something you are doing for yourself. You may face resistance from your family at first. However, when you begin to heal yourself, you also usher in healing into your family system. Therefore, you are also doing it for your family and future generations. You are part of their healing. You will pass down medicine instead of trauma to the next generation.

MESSAGES IN OUR VEINS

Intergenerational trauma is not just a feeling or vague buzzword everyone is talking about. According to Dr. Galit Atlas, a psychoanalyst and author of *Emotional Inheritance: A Therapist, Her Patients, and the Legacy of Trauma*, who we become is based on what we experienced, as well as what our parents and ancestors experienced.[1] There are emotional markers in our molecules that tell our body how to express the trauma through various genetic expressions. The genetic markers in our DNA are transcribed with information from our mothers' DNA, which is full of information from their mothers' DNA, and so on. It is almost like a memory carried in our genes from one generation to the next. The genetic markers are informants more than determinants or catalysts.

Intergenerational trauma is defined as trauma that gets passed down from those who directly experienced the trauma to subsequent generations. It can begin with a traumatic event affecting an individual or multiple family members, or collective trauma affecting larger communities. Parents may transmit genetic vulnerabilities triggered by their own traumatic experiences, which may also impact their parenting styles. Some genetic vulnerabilities passed down due to trauma include higher risk for depression, anxiety, substance abuse, emotional dysregulation, and relational challenges. People who have experienced trauma have difficulty bonding and creating healthy emotional attachments with others, including their partners and children.

Children form their sense of identity, safety, and attachment styles through how they were raised by their primary caregivers. Many times, we mimic our parents' behaviors and navigate our relationships based on how we relate to our parents and their parenting styles. Our coping mechanisms are skills or behaviors we develop to try to avoid or fix our parents' abuse, anger, depression, neglect, and other hurtful behaviors. The relationship between a parent with unprocessed trauma and their child, who inherited genetic vulnerabilities brought on by said trauma, can be challenging. Parents with unprocessed trauma may have a hard time expressing, feeling, and regulating their emotions. They may not have the tools to meet their own needs, which impairs their ability to meet their child's needs. This perpetuates a cycle of neglect or abuse and increases the risk of the child experiencing trauma, mental health issues, substance abuse tendencies, and difficulty creating healthy, safe attachments.

When trauma is so deeply woven into the infrastructure of our family systems, it is almost impossible not to weave it into how we love. Sometimes we confuse the two. We treat trauma as if it were another family member. Many of us call that bond love. We call it being a tight-knit family. With each generation, the cord feels tighter, and the weight of intergenerational trauma becomes more suffocating. We will continue gasping for air until someone breaks the cord.

Most women in my family carried shame, rejection, and a sense of worthlessness in their DNA. They experienced, witnessed, and remembered trauma around their bodies, sexuality, womanhood, and relationships. Many of them grew up fearing or chasing men. They grew up fearing and hating their bodies. They believed they were less worthy of respect and dignity simply because they were women. They didn't receive acceptance or healthy messages around their sexuality, only shame. The fear of being exploited, the reality of poverty, and the trauma of racism braided together created a crowning state of stress. This became my emotional inheritance. Eventually, I started living and believing it myself. I was receiving the messages—abuse, machismo, and shame—they received from them directly, from my DNA, and from the environment around me.

Oftentimes when we think of hereditary illnesses or ailments being passed down from one generation to the other, we mainly think of physical diseases or sickness. However, some of the most harmful hereditary illnesses and wounds are emotional and psychological. Many of us hold the pain of shame, rejection, and neglect. We inherit these deep-rooted messages which tell us we are unlovable and unwanted. There is no over-the-counter remedy for these types of ailments. As I've said, sanar es un proceso. Any wound is difficult to treat when it is invisible—when we do not have the words or tools to identify it. Looking into our past allows us to bring light into our present and make more informed choices about our future.

Before we proceed, I want you to take a quiet moment for you. Visualize yourself holding a candle. Take a moment to feel the warmth of the flame in your hands. This is your light. All yours. No one can take it from you. You will be bringing this light to the dark. Your dark and your shadows. Your fears and your wounds. They are nothing to be afraid of. They are simply parts of you that need medicine, cariño, y mucho amor. Those are the parts of you that perhaps have been neglected and need un apapacho. We will be bringing that to them now: medicina y apapachos para tus heridas. You are entering with your power, with your softness, with your tenderness, with care, with awareness, with consciousness, with tools, with ancestral wisdom, with intention. Respira.

Now, still in this visualization, picture the many other women and beings also reading this book and walking this journey with you. Picture their light, their flame in their hands. Picture all of us bringing our lights together in the middle. Our light is powerful as a collective. We are bringing in so much medicine to the depths of the intergenerational wounds that tie many of us together. There is so much power in the work you are doing. Que no se nos olvide. This work is for the greater good and collective liberation. No estás sola. Estamos contigo.

Ahora, picture yourself walking into the dark. It is familiar. You are safe now. You do not live there anymore. Your home is in the light. You know the way out. You have light with you and around you. You are not alone. You are not the scared child who was abandoned there. You are an adult now. Eres una guerrera. You are going in with a purpose. You are going in to bring love and healing. You will not stay there; you are just visiting. This is you loving yourself, your inner niña, and your future self. This is intergenerational healing. Lo estás haciendo, Badass Bonita.

You are an active participant in the intergenerational healing and collective liberation of your people—our people. The way you love yourself is directly connected to the collective's liberation. The words you speak and the messages we pass on will impact generations to come. Eres poderosa, mujer.

Some questions to consider include:

How will you use your voice to usher in liberation, healing, and strength?

What messages are you uprooting?

What cycles will stop with you?

What messages are you planting like seeds in your garden?

Breathe in and acknowledge the strength within you. Eres luz. Eres una guerrera. Eres una Badass Bonita. There is revolutionary love running through your veins. There was a moment when I realized that the messages that I will pass on to the next generation had to be messages of love and liberation.

GENOGRAM

A genogram is a graphic depiction of how different family members are biologically, legally, and emotionally related to one another from one generation to the next. As a therapeutic family mapping tool, genograms help us understand the intergenerational cycles and relationships between family systems. Recognizing these patterns often helps families avoid repeating them and transmitting them to future generations.

In a genogram, each of the symbols represents a person, their sexuality, gender, and life experience. From divorces to miscarriages, the genogram not only describes the relationships each family member has with one another like a traditional family tree, but the life events that may impact each relationship. The genogram symbols and interpersonal interactions relationship legend help us name and understand the various dynamics between family members. We can observe emotional distance, affection, abusive patterns, and unhealthy attachments throughout the generations.

Visit my website at https://brownbadassbonita.com/pages/therapy-resources, to see what a genogram looks like. There, you'll find examples of the various symbols, and also my own genogram. This will help you begin to understand what the different relationships and connections are. On a folded piece of paper, begin to draw the different branches of your ancestral tree according to the symbols that best describe their life experience, starting with the most senior members.

For example, you can begin by adding your grandparents on both your maternal and paternal sides. The symbol for a woman is a circle and the symbol for a man is a square. So, if your grandparents were a heterosexual couple on your paternal and maternal side, add a circle and a square on both sides. Then add the lines depicting their relational connection: married, widowed, divorced, cut off, close, etc. You can add the markers for emotional abuse, substance abuse, etc., if those were present within this generation and their relationship to each other. There are also markers for immigration, miscarriages, illness, and living in two cultures. If there has been a death in your grandparents' generation, you can mark it by putting an "X" inside their symbol. The more life-changing events that have happened in your family, the more connecting lines you may have.

In my genogram, my mother and father both come from mothers who were emotionally and physically abusive and absent fathers they are cut off from. My parents are not together and their distant relationship is portrayed by a dotted line. Both remarried and had children from their second marriages, and my mom is on to her third marriage. Going through these branches, you can see the relational pattern of emotional abuse and paternal cutoff being passed down on both sides of my family.

Having a visual representation of what your family has been through can provide a deeper level of understanding of your background and how necessary the act of healing can be. Remember that the genogram is not meant to be perfect. It's not about getting every symbol for every person right. The goal of the genogram is to see the ripple effect. It's to see the way trauma travels, like vines on a branch connecting each part of your family tree. Many times, people that do this exercise find the number of squiggly lines in their chart overwhelming or upsetting. They want justice, they want accountability, they sit on the anger that comes from knowing so many people have survived very fucked-up circumstances. Others find their genogram missing big chunks of their family, their absence a visual reminder of abandonment, pain, or familial outcasts. Usually, there are more lines than people, and the hurt and pain that connects them outweighs everything.

Seeing how interconnected trauma can be in your family may be scary. You may think, *I don't want to become a squiggly line for someone else.* That awareness is what brought you to this healing work, and that awareness can be your tool to break the cycle, if you choose to do so. Chances are the people in your genogram wanted justice for what was done to them. Chances are they want the same things you do, like peace, accountability, and acknowledgement. Your healing gets to be a voice for them. You get to be a voice for them.

Approaching this exercise with cariño can mean taking it slow, working at your own pace, going on walks, or taking breaks. There may be times when you feel the weight of the intergenerational trauma within your family system. Holding their stories and learning about all that your family has lived through te puede apachurrar el corazón.

BIRTH ORDER THEORY

Birth order refers to the successive way children appear in a family line and the personality traits and behaviors that can develop because of the expectations and treatment associated with each rank. When mapping out your genogram, it is important to consider how birth order may also be a contributing factor to a family member's actions or experiences. An only child, for instance, may appear more confident and mature for their age because they tend to spend more time with adults and they don't have to share parental attention with siblings. As a result, they can struggle with the concept of sharing, or may appear arrogant. An eldest sibling can come across as responsible and controlling, since they are often tasked with taking care of the rest of the family. Meanwhile, the youngest sibling can appear more outgoing and carefree since they tend to experience extra attention from their parents, or are raised with a different, often more flexible, set of expectations.

Many firstborn, first-generation Latinas have to grow up quickly and become an adjacent part to the parenting unit in the family system. We are often made responsible for ourselves, our siblings, and our parents. Most of the cycle breakers I've met are firstborn Latinas who are finally taking care of themselves and nurturing their mental health. There is a loneliness (and sometimes even guilt) that comes with being the first. I always say that being firstborn, first-gen Latinas should be something we're allowed to put on our résumes!

When I added a more cultural consciousness to the birth order theory, I felt seen and held. I'm able to hold a more complete understanding of my family system. When I was following the "eldest Latina daughter" rules of overachievement, people pleasing, and self-sacrifice I was praised and put on a pedestal. When I began to heal and develop an identity of my own outside the role set out for me, I was shamed, ostracized, and made to feel like a disgrace. I went from being the first golden child to being treated as if I was purposefully making my family less and less proud. The more "me" I felt, the less accepted and celebrated I became within my family system.

Not only is it necessary to consider the impact of birth order, cultural values, and systemic oppression on our family systems, but it is also essential to understand the impact of trauma. Adding a more trauma-informed lens to your understanding of your family system can help your healing journey by providing a more conscious, compassionate, proactive, and preventive awareness. Trauma awareness and consciousness is necessary for second-order changes—otherwise known as long-lasting, systemic change—to family systems. Second-order change comes when you do things differently and, therefore, get different results, which changes the path the family was previously on. For example, if the family was on a course of repeating traumatic behaviors and patterns, and one person changes this path by going to therapy, raising their awareness, understanding the sources of the trauma, and consciously choosing not to repeat the pattern or engage in behaviors which cause trauma, they break the cycle of trauma and change the path of the family. This is second-order change.[2]

According to the research, these are additional factors that influence the development of our personalities:

- Biological: Children inherit many traits and features from their parents. These include intelligence, courage, and physical features. Resistance is literally in our blood.
- Social: We learn behaviors and thought patterns from observing our parents, community, and peers.
- Cultural: Our culture consciously and unconsciously influences us to adopt traits which uphold the culture's beliefs and norms.
- Physical Environment: An individual's surroundings often have a direct impact on the development of their personalities. For example, the personalities of those growing up in a rural area are often very different from those living in an urban environment. Growing up in East LA is very different from growing up in rural Wisconsin.
- Situational: As a child grows, they face different situations, which help them adapt and change aspects of their personalities. This could include meeting new friends, experiencing trauma, or welcoming a new sibling.[3]

As we begin to dissect the intersections and layers of our identities within our family systems, we can see the complexity we must navigate through as we begin our journey of self-discovery and liberation. We are operating within a family system operating within a larger system of oppression and oftentimes with internalized oppression as well. The values to which our family subscribes, consciously or unconsciously, impact the whole family system. They may benefit some and oppress others. We are born into these systems, which have been operating for generations. We must raise our awareness to dismantle these oppressive systems.

ACES:
ADVERSE CHILDHOOD EXPERIENCES

The first time I learned about ACEs was during training at Mission Hope, a shelter for women recovering from homelessness, addiction, and domestic violence in Seattle. I was a case manager working with unhoused women in recovery from addiction and domestic violence. Most of the case managers were in recovery themselves or had experienced some sort of trauma. During our lunch break from the training session, a group of us sat on the same side of the cafeteria table, backs covered and with a clear view of the exit, all of us collectively hypervigilant in case some shit hit the fan.

Once we returned to the session, we were given an assessment that measured how much childhood trauma we experienced. The results of the assessment were called an ACE score, or an Adverse Childhood Experience score. When the training facilitators had us share our scores, most of us had between between six and nine out of ten, indicating moderate-to-high levels of trauma. The only person that scored a zero was the director of Mission Hope. With our trauma scores in hand, I started seeing the adults in the room differently. We were once children who went through really difficult situations. We were now adults with scars, wounds, and a desire to heal. I was in a room full of survivors and warriors.

ACEs are potentially traumatic events that occur during childhood. The Centers for Disease Control and Prevention (CDC) and Kaiser Permanente conducted the first ACEs study covering the years 1995 to 1997. They asked more than 17,000 adults about negative childhood experiences, including emotional abuse, physical abuse, sexual abuse, neglect, parental separation, substance abuse, incarceration, violence, and mental illness.[4]

Most of the participants had experienced at least one ACE. About 20 percent of the participants reported three or more ACEs. Researchers linked ACE exposure to a higher likelihood of negative health and behavioral challenges later in life, such as heart disease, diabetes, and premature death. Higher ACE scores also suggest increased risk for mental illness, including depression, alcoholism, and post-traumatic stress disorder (PTSD). The results suggest that kids who have experienced high ACEs may be more likely to perpetuate abuse, behave aggressively, or be revictimized in the future. This also impacts an individual's behavior in school, their likelihood of unemployment, as well as higher risk of smoking and drug use. Recently, the CDC found that at least half of the top leading causes of death, including respiratory illnesses, heart disease, cancer, and suicide, are associated with higher ACEs.[5]

According to the ACE study, there are ten different types of adverse childhood experiences. These are divided into three categories: abuse, neglect, and household dysfunction. The assessment asks you questions pertaining to each kind of abuse and marks a point for each type of adverse childhood experience you personally lived through.

The assessment asks questions such as:
Before your 18th birthday, did a parent or adult in the household often or very often…

- Swear at you, insult you, humiliate you, or make you feel unsafe, afraid, or fearful due to their aggressive or violent behavior?
- Push, grab, slap, or throw something at you, or ever hit you so hard that you had marks or were injured?
- Touch or fondle your body or have you touch their body in a sexual way? Attempt or have oral, anal, or vaginal intercourse with you?

Did you often or very often:

- Feel like no one in your family loved you or thought you were important or special, or feel like your family didn't look out for each other, feel close, or support each other?
- Lack enough food to eat, have to wear dirty clothes, or feel like no one was there to protect you, or have parents that were too drunk or high to take care of you?
- Lose a biological parent through divorce, abandonment, or other reasons?
- Experience violence through pushing, grabbing, slapping, or throwing things or receiving violent behavior, or were threatened with a gun or knife?
- Live with anyone who was a problem drinker, alcoholic, or abused drugs?

- Feel depressed or mentally ill or attempted/committed suicide?
- Have a caregiver go to prison?

Toxic, chronic stress is the underlying mechanism by which ACEs manifest themselves externally and impact an individual's physical, psychological, and mental wellness. Toxic stress in the body interrupts or impedes the healthy development of neural, immune, and hormonal systems, especially among children. I imagine our inner niñas growing up with toxic stress in their little bodies. I grieve what the trauma took from us. We carry our grandmother's trauma in our veins. Awareness of adverse childhood experiences helps us protect our inner niñas from being exposed to the same trauma. Our adult selves can then use this information to take care of our future selves. I also picture our mamis, tías, and family members with these memories of adverse experiences running through their veins and their roots. If they were not able to heal these wounds, they passed them on and now they are running through our veins. You were probably at a higher risk to experience trauma yourself if you had parents or caregivers who had unresolved trauma. This is how the cycle continues until we choose to end it by healing and doing things differently. In order to heal, you must know what needs healing, what is bleeding, and what medicine will help the wound.

This is a lot of information, pero it is meant to help you understand your roots and what needs to be uprooted. See it not as something to fear, but as you shining a light onto your past so that you can sow seeds for a better future for yourself and future generations. Now that you have an increased awareness, you have more power to know what you're working with, what you can change, and what you can prevent. It gives you more awareness of the areas that need healing and extra care in your life. It can increase your motivation to care for your mind and body, as well as your emotional and spiritual well-being.

Understanding the roots and family tree you come from is just as important as understanding the soil you were born into. The more we understand, the more we can heal. Take your time to understand your family tree's roots (history, trauma, stories, culture, values, beliefs), the trunk (the values which uphold the functioning of your family system), the branches (the people who make up the family tree), and the flora (the fruit or foliage your tree is bearing, including children, cycles, messages, etc.). Where and who you come from is important. They may not be pretty or perfect, but they are valuable. This is information about who you are and who you are becoming. Honor each piece, cada hoja, cada raíz, cada persona. Take a moment to look at yourself and your family con ojos de amor y compasión. You have been through a lot, individually and collectively. Think of the things you overcame as a family and the wars that were fought before you were even born. Look at the scars and battle wounds. Mira dónde están floreciendo las cicatrices. Trace the patterns and cycles down to the roots and see the picture they paint. What are they trying to tell you? Where are the wounds still bleeding? Trace the roots and see where they are connected to you. Think about your healing and what you want to pass down. Think of the cycles you'd like to break and the wounds you'd like to heal. Send love and gratitude to your family system for all they did and how hard they tried, for not giving up, and for doing their best with what they had. Send compassion and forgiveness for the wounds they caused, what they did, couldn't or didn't do, what they didn't or couldn't give, and for passing on their wounds. Take a moment to hold yourself and thank yourself for doing this work. Think of yourself as a branch on the family tree and tell yourself:

"Pronto vamos a estar floreciendo."

Reflexiones

The following exercises are meant to help us reflect on how our ancestors have blessed, harmed, taught, and paved the road for us. Make sure to leave room to grieve, rage, burn sage, cry, and feel all the emotions that come up as you process this.

Make a list of the blessings, strengths, and resilience you've inherited from your family members.

Write a letter of gratitude to your family for the battles they fought and the blessings they passed on. Thank them for doing the best they could with what they had.

Take note of which cycles you wish to break or not pass down. Take note of which mistakes you are going to learn from to make different choices.

THE MADRE WOUND

When I was younger, I'd watch everything my mami did, listened to everything she said, and trailed her every step.

If she didn't like blueberries, neither did I. If she hated cats, I did too, no questions asked. Some people believed in la Virgen de

Guadalupe, yet I worshiped mi mami. My mami was my main educator on beauty, womanhood, and love. I memorized what she told me, feeling like it was my job not only to be like her, but to protect her and make sure she was always happy. I followed her until it hurt, and even then, I kept going. Her words were my medicine and poison, my map to this world, and all that I knew. They were everything. She was my everything.

The summer I told mi mami her boyfriend had sexually abused me for years since I was nine years old, she got mad at me. She began treating me as if I had ruined her life once again. There was hate in her emerald eyes. I broke the silence that was protecting him. In turn, she broke the bond between us in order to protect him. She blamed me for ruining the family. Not him. Me. I ruined the family when I spoke up about her man abusing me. All of a sudden, I was the villain and the victim. It felt like I was more her enemy than her daughter.

As the years progressed, this sentiment deepened. The wound was wide open and there was no stopping the bleeding. We kept fighting over the abuse. She kept telling me to get over it. I needed to stop being the victim, which in her eyes also made me the villain. I needed to simply move on and let her go back to living her life. Even though we stopped talking about it to maintain a semblance of peace, the wound didn't go away. I began to distance myself because being close to mi mami hurt me. I needed her, yet her presence and her absence hurt me. I didn't know it then, but these were moments where she was fighting her own internal and intergenerational battles. These are battles many women in our lineage had to fight. They won when they broke the silence, protected those who needed protecting, and held abusers accountable. Unfortunately, many women betrayed themselves and their daughters when they kept quiet in order to keep the peace and protect their men. I didn't know how to make sense of it. Sometimes, I still don't.

There were times she'd tell me, "I wish I wasn't your mother!" or "From now on, don't consider me your mother. I am done!"

She finished that conversation with a "¡Dios te bendiga!" and stopped talking to me for months. There was rage, jealousy, and resentment. Many times, I asked myself, how is it that this woman who birthed me could hate me so much?

Our relationship with our mothers is a very formative one, whether good, bad, or nonexistent. For many of us it is the first relationship we have. Generally speaking, our lives depend on this relationship. Depending on the closeness and culture, our relationship with our mothers is indispensable. We are raised to be close to our mamis, even if our mamis hurt us.

The mother wound prevents the establishment of a secure, loving attachment between mother and child.[6] It is an ache and a desperate longing for the mother's love you wished for, but never got. Mi mami longed for her mami and her mami longed for her mami and her mami longed for her mami. Our mamis were not taught how to love themselves or other women. They were taught to shrink and silence themselves and other women. They teach what they were taught. They teach what they know. It is a chain of broken mamis with broken hearts, longing for the softness and gentleness of maternal love and care. It is a state of constant grieving for a mother that may never come. Many of our childhoods were filled with this longing and with us doing everything we could to somehow get an ounce of love and approval from our mothers.

This wound is usually a manifestation of a mother not meeting her child's emotional needs. There is a need we all have for love, care, and safety. There is a wound when that need isn't met, especially from our primary caregiver. Mothers who wound their children were often wounded by their own mothers. They usually have unmet needs themselves and are not able to give love in the way their child needs because they didn't receive the love they needed as a children. It is a dark cycle of broken hearts breaking the next generation's, and the next, down the ancestral line.

There is a particular type of mother wound that is characteristic of narcissistic mothers and that we need to address. Narcissism is a personality disorder which must be assessed and diagnosed by a professional. However, there are certain narcissistic tendencies we see commonly across cultures. Mothers with narcissistic tendencies tend to treat their children, most commonly their daughters, as an extension of themselves, as a threat, as someone they manipulate to control and maintain power. Other behaviors commonly seen in mothers with narcissistic tendencies include:

- Shaming you
- Displaying jealousy toward you
- Becoming enraged at any perceived threat to her superiority
- Invalidating or guilt-tripping you
- Violating or pushing your boundaries
- Playing favorites with their children or making them compete for her love, acceptance, and attention
- Making herself the center of conversations and situations in general
- Putting you down to elevate her self-esteem[7]

There are long-term wounds that come from having a mother with narcissistic tendencies that include:

Belief in Conditional Love. Mothers with narcissistic tendencies instill a belief in their daughters that love is conditional. They usually provide love when they want to and on their terms. They do not make their daughters feel like they deserve love simply for being themselves. These mothers' ups and downs and unpredictable demonstrations of love can lead to their children's emotional disorientation. This in turn can lead to disorganized attachment, difficulty maintaining healthy relationships, and low self-esteem. This form of conditional love leaves daughters feeling like they have to perform in certain ways or abide by certain rules (even if it means sacrificing their own wants, needs, and well-being) in order to receive love and acceptance.

Appearances Are Everything. How you appear is very important to a mother with narcissistic tendencies, because it is a reflection of her. Especially if you are seen as an extension of her, your success, appearance, public persona, and achievements are imperative to her. This puts pressure on the daughter to be valued and validated by others. Her sense of self is dependent on others' perceptions of her, not allowing her to be her authentic self. There is a pressure to be who your mother wants you to be—or else. You do things thinking of her. You become who she wants you to be. You say what will make her happy. You like what she likes. You are at her service. You live for her and to be loved by her.

Accepting Mistreatment. If your mother was emotionally abusive and/or manipulative, you learned from an early age to accept mistreatment and correlate it with love.

Abuse and manipulation may have been the norm for you as a child and, therefore, you may have interpreted them as normal behaviors and treatment within loving relationships. As an adult, you have to learn that manipulation and abuse are not part of healthy relationships. Love and abuse cannot coexist. It doesn't matter who they are, if they abuse you—it isn't love. You deserve better. Mereces amor bonito, no maltratos.

Regularly Blaming Yourself. Accountability is really hard for narcissistic mothers. They usually blame you for their problems. You learn to take the blame over and over. This can lead to an unstable sense of self. You start doubting yourself and believing everything is really your fault. You internalize this feeling of worthlessness. So often, none of it was your fault, mujer. Yet you carried so much for so long when you were far too small to even know what was happening. You carried things you were never meant to carry. It is time to release.

People Pleasing. Feeling like you are constantly living to please your mother and meet her needs can lead you to develop people-pleasing tendencies as a way to receive love and acceptance. You may learn to neglect your own needs or constantly feel like a burden to others. Constantly focusing your energy on meeting someone else's needs can lead to you developing a core belief that your needs don't deserve to be met. You don't learn what it feels like for someone to take care of you and support you. You don't know how to do that for yourself or receive it from someone else. You grow up believing your main purpose is to please others and meet their needs.

Chasing Love. Lacking a sense of safety due to your mother's neglect, abuse, or emotional maltreatment can lead to insecure attachments which will have you chasing and questioning your relationships. When you do not receive the love you need from your primary caregiver(s), there is a high chance you will spend most of your life looking for and chasing that love. We must learn to give it to ourselves. The neglect and lack of empathy often displayed by mothers with narcissistic tendencies can leave us feeling like there is something missing and/or wrong with us.[8]

We often chase people because we believe no one will want to stay with us. This sense of worthlessness and rejection can often lead us to chase external validation as well. If you find someone who wants to have a committed relationship with you, you may find yourself needing constant reassurance and validation. There may be an internalized fear of them not actually loving you, because you didn't feel loved by your mother. These things may feel frightening because you may be unfamiliar with the feeling of someone loving you for you, unconditionally and consistently. This is intimately and ultimately tied to how we were loved growing up. We must develop a secure attachment with ourselves in order to have a secure attachment with others and stop chasing after love and external validation. Ya tienes todo lo que necesitas: ¡te tienes a ti, mujer!

The wounds caused by mothers with narcissistic tendencies are deep and long-lasting. They cling to us like vines with thorns. If some of these behaviors or beliefs resonate with you and your relationship with your mother, I recommend taking time to learn more about narcissism from research and a professional. Most importantly, to take time to validate your experience and give yourself compassion for having been through such a challenging relationship. Relationships with mothers with narcissistic tendencies are complicated and often very harmful. Although you cannot control them or make them change, you can heal and recover. You have the tools and the medicine now. Do it for you and your inner niña. Do it for you and your future self.

La verdadera medicina for the mother wound is mothering that inner niña that grew up needing the love and apapachos her mami wasn't able to give her. Loving that inner niña and holding her close. Let her know you will take care of her and give her all the love she needs. Learn to listen to your own voice, the one they told you to silence.

It took me a long time to realize it doesn't matter what I do or who I am—it won't ever fill the ache for my mother in my heart. After years of rage, resentment, and angry letters addressed to my mother—I was finally able to forgive her. The bitterness was getting too heavy—like veneno in my veins. It was getting in the way of me learning to love me. Some say forgiveness is also medicine, not for the person who hurt you, but for you. Set yourself free with the realization that you are the one that deserves peace.

So, I decided to release the rage in order to embrace me. This allowed me to see my mother as a woman who also had a mother wound. Her inner niña also just wanted to be held and loved by her mami. It did not excuse her actions or lack of accountability. It did not stop the bleeding, but it freed me up enough to continue the healing. Seeing my mother's wounds did not heal them nor did it heal mine, but it offered me the sufficient compassion and understanding to continue with my own journey. I was able to see her story with compassion while choosing to write a different story for myself.

I am choosing to write a love story between me and my inner niña and the woman I am becoming.

I am choosing to write a love story about myself and my soul.

Reflexiones

I am healing for me.

I am healing for mi mami and her mami.

I am healing for my inner niña, my daughters, and their daughters.

- *Imagine your mami's inner niña. What did she need to hear growing up? What are some words that she may have needed her mami to tell her that may have healed her heart?*

- *Imagine your mother as a young girl. What would you tell her that you think she needed to hear?*

- *What are the things you and your mami have in common? What are the things that make you different? How can you hold and differentiate both of your identities, needs, and experiences? How are you and your mother similar? Are the qualities that make you different celebrated or criticized?*

- *What are the wounds you received from your mother? What is the medicine you received from her? How will you mother your inner niña to tend to those wounds? Think about when you needed your mother the most. Did she support you in the way you wanted her to? How can you bring medicine to these wounds?*

Chapter 3

Mensajitos in Our Garden

Mujer, ¿cuáles son las semillas plantadas en tu jardín? ¿Quién las plantó? What seeds are planted in your garden and who planted them there? Los mensajes que crecimos escuchando are like plants that we kept watering. Los mensajes que recibimos y creímos mientras crecíamos son como semillas we kept watering. Now they are plantitas or weeds growing in our garden, one of the most prominent ones being: "Calladita te ves más bonita." Most of these messages were passed down from one generation to the next. Nuestras mamis nos dicen lo que sus mamis les dijeron porque sus mamis les dijeron lo mismo, and so on and so on. We receive them and let them grow within us as truths because our mami's words guide us and sustain us as we grow. Cuando somos niñas, we don't stop and question what our mami tells us. Her words are what we hold on to in order to make sense of this world. We drink them como si fueran medicina, unaware that sometimes these words wound us from the inside. Algunos de estos mensajes son semillas that should never have been planted in our garden. These messages have grown deep roots in our garden and impacted our perspective and experience of womanhood, motherhood, family, identity, relationships, love, sex, and self. Most of these messages are rooted in machismo, misogyny, racism, colonialism, and systems of oppression. They must be uprooted. These are the messages that wound us and have wounded many men and women in our families. These intergenerational messages point to places where we still need healing and liberation. Las mujeres de nuestra familia are our first and most enduring educators. Nos enseñan con sus palabras, con sus miradas, con sus manitas arrugadas. Nos enseñan cómo vestirnos, sentarnos y comportarnos. Nos enseñan lo que les enseñaron. Nos enseñan lo que saben y nos dan todo lo que tienen; trauma, pain, and poison included. De estos mensajes we will learn to make magia y medicina porque eso es lo que somos: mujeres, magia, medicina.

These intergenerational messages point to places where we still need healing and liberation.

This is the unearthing. The beginning of uproot. Yet the process of uprooting is often a painful one that takes years and looks different for each garden: each individual and each family system. Pero de alguna manera se tiene que empezar.

As we explore these messages, imagine you are entering your garden. Enter con cariño and curiosity. You will be walking through your garden exploring the weeds and flowers that are growing there. You get to decide which ones you want to keep watering and which ones you'd like to uproot. Then, you get to plant new seeds: mensajes de amor y liberación.

The following sections hold common messages that were planted into many of our gardens. These include semillitas telling us about our bodies, beauty, sex lives, etc. Oftentimes, our mami told us these things because her mami told her and her mami told her.

BODY

"Si engordo, me mato."

When I was in high school, my mom told me she'd kill herself if she ever got fat. By then, my eating disorder was well on its way. Eating two Cup Noodles for breakfast and any snacks I could find became my regular. At the Salvation Army, I bought a baggy checkered dress that was a mix between a mumu and something you'd buy at a Cracker Barrel. My self-esteem at that point was low and I felt the need to constantly cover myself.

One day, I wore the dress to Target, where the cashier happened to be my Tita's friend. Later that evening, my Tita called my mom yelling, saying her friend thought I was pregnant. "¡Está tan gorda y panzona que ya piensan que está embarazada! ¡Tiene que bajar de peso! Tiene que adelgazar."

From that day forward I put myself on a diet. There were times I'd work out until I passed out. I became obsessed with losing weight. By the time I was in eighth grade, all my bones were protruding. My mom would yell at me for not eating enough, forcing me to finish my plate, but I'd always work off the calories or pop a laxative.

They didn't know I started eating to cope with the abuse. The abuse got worse during the summer vacations, when my siblings went to live with their dad and I stayed home alone. I ate to cope with the loneliness and the shame. I felt there was definitely something wrong with me and my body. I must be doing something wrong. I wanted it to stop, but I didn't know how. So I ate in an attempt to comfort myself, but also to change my body. There wasn't much I had control over. I felt dirty and so unlovable. I had control over what I ate and what my body looked like.

My mom and my stepdad kept warning me about men staring at my body and treating me differently once my body started changing. The man in my home definitely did. So, maybe if I changed my body, it would protect me. Maybe if I hid it beneath the ugliest plaid floral dress, I'd be a little bit safer from their hungry eyes. So I ate, and I ate. I had nothing else to do. Until that comment from the woman at Target. Esa pinche vieja chismosa has no idea what her words did to me that summer.

I became obsessed. The shame consumed me and took over my life. I was ashamed of my body: what was happening to it, what it looked like, what people were saying about it, how men were looking at it. I was certain there was not one lovable thing about my body. Everyone was warning me about my body, and not one person said a loving thing toward it. My body was full of shame inside and out. Shame makes us feel like we are unlovable. Shame lathered my skin like sweat on a hot summer day. Now, I had to change my body again so that the lady at Target would stop telling people I looked pregnant. Most importantly, I did it so that my mami and Tita wouldn't be ashamed of me. I also wanted them to stop shaming my body. I did that just fine, thank you.

Hearing my mother say that she'd rather die than be fat confirmed I was doing the right thing. I was torturing and shrinking my body. Food and exercise became my punishment and all I lived for. I'd spend hours looking at my body and hyper analyzing all the "faults." I'd be so harsh on myself. The only things I'd tell myself about my body were venomous.

Eating disorders aren't really spoken about in our cultura. This is often dismissed and regarded as a white girl thing. Even though

recent studies show similarities in prevalence, risk factors, symptom-
ology, and psychopathology in eating disorders between white girls
and Latinas[1]. Often, Latinas don't know how to talk about their eat-
ing habits, beliefs around food and body image, relationship with
food and health, etc. There is too much shame and a lack of knowl-
edge. We don't seek out help or treatment, not knowing where to
start, or facing accessibility issues. Even with telenovela episodes
highlighting the issue, like in *La Rosa de Guadalupe*, there are still
complexities with the way body issues are treated in many Latine fam-
ilies. With a large emphasis on food, many Latinas find themselves
caught in a similar back and forth effect of appearing ungrateful for
not eating everything served to them, criticized for making differ-
ent food choices, or judged for embracing their appearance. Coupled
with the expectations of machismo and marianismo, which prioritize
women's appearance and aesthetics as functions of patriarchy, many
Latinas experience a feeling of hopelessness in constantly striving for,
but never achieving, standards that seem to always change. No matter
what we do, we get in trouble for being muy flacas or muy gordas.

Not once did I hear a woman in my family say something loving
about their body. Ni una vez. This is heartbreaking. I'm here to break
that cycle. So are you. May the women (and men) in our families see
us eating without shame, treating our bodies con cariño, and simply
loving ourselves as we are. Imagine you saw the mujeres in your fam-
ily loving themselves and feeling free and comfortable in their bod-
ies. Imagine you saw them smile and speak kind things when they
looked in the mirror. Instead, many of us saw our mamis frown when
they looked at themselves in the mirror. Our abuelas shied away
from the camera porque decían que eran feas. They never learned to
call themselves beautiful or see themselves con ojos de amor. You get
to be that woman in your family.

Reflexiones

- *What is your relationship with your body like? Is it like the relationship the women in your family have with their bodies?*

- *How have messages about your body impacted your inner niña? What messages would you tell her now about her body?*

- *Write your body a love poem.*

BEAUTY

"Calladita te ves más bonita."

"Las guapas se aguantan."

"No salgas greñuda y sin arreglarte."

"No seas fodonga."

"A las feas nadie las quiere."

Too many niñas grow up believing they are most beautiful when they are quiet. This is a seed that must be uprooted. It is a lie. We are not most beautiful when we are quiet. We are most beautiful when we love ourselves. We are most beautiful when we step into our power. This is a message that feeds the roots of the many branches in our family tree. In many Latine families, beauty is a goal to be achieved, through mannerisms and aesthetic. Together with the physical expectations many Latinas work within, beauty standards are aspirational because beauty signifies goodness and value as a person. Individual families can define beauty by measures like lighter skin tones, European features, weight, or hair texture. In addition to these tangible attributes, beauty can be found in how compliant a woman is: If she doesn't talk back, she is beautiful. If she does things without question, she is beautiful. If she does as she is told, she is beautiful.

True beauty is something we need to define and find within ourselves. I refuse to be one more woman who does not find beauty within herself. I will find it and embody my beauty. I will not be afraid to be beautiful. I will not apologize for my beauty. Me ha costado demasiado encontrarla y no la voy a soltar. It has cost me too much to find it and I will not lose it again. When you see me, you will see a queer greñuda amándose. They often teach us to aguantarnos. They rarely teach us to amarnos. Porque cuando nos amamos, we see ourselves con ojos de amor and we become unstoppable, untameable, unfuckwithable.

We are taught to aguantar in order to be beautiful, in order to be loved, in order to be accepted. Aguantar feels like shutting your eyes tight, teeth gritted, fists knotted, and betraying what your body, mind, and corazón tell you they need. I've seen too many women aguantándose. Nos aguantamos because we are taught that being beautiful is one of the most important things we can do. Beauty is what many women depended on in order to survive. Beauty is what got them married, and married is what made them successful, accepted, and respected. If you weren't beautiful or trying to be beautiful era casi casi una condena: una mujer fracasada. If you were not trying to catch the attention of men or appearing beautiful for the male gaze, you were just not doing it right. It wasn't until my adulthood that I began creating my own definition of beauty. I am slowly unlearning the beauty standards I grew up abiding by and learning to create my own definition of beauty. When do I feel and look most beautiful? What makes other people beautiful in my eyes?

Our silence does not equal beauty. This is a weapon of oppression. Fuck that, mija! Usa tu voz. Grita. Canta. Cuenta tu historia. Tu voz es parte de tu belleza. Your voice adds to your beauty. There was a time I was looking at myself in the mirror naked and I started thinking of how I was lied to my whole life about what made me beautiful. In that moment of nakedness, I found the beauty and strength within me. I felt most beautiful when I first said "No" to my abuser. I was most beautiful when I broke my silence and told my whole story for the first time. I was sobbing between words. My voice was shaking. I was being the bravest I'd ever been. I was beauty embodied. I was most beautiful when I began reciting my poetry to a crowd of women and niñas. I was most beautiful when I gave my first TEDx talk. I am most beautiful when I make loving choices for myself, use my voice, and step into my power. So are you.

Our beauty does not have to come accompanied by pain. Neither does love.

Reflexiones

- *What is your definition of beauty? How would you describe someone who is beautiful? What does a beautiful person look like to you? How do they act? What do they value?*

- *What are the parts of yourself that you love? What makes you beautiful?*

- *When are the moments in which you have felt most beautiful? Who was the first person in your life that you considered beautiful? Describe them.*

- *What is preventing you from seeing and embodying your beauty? What message have you been staying quiet about? How would you feel if you finally let it out?*

LOVE AND CODEPENDENT
RELATIONSHIPS

Earlier, I described how, when I got married, everyone started treating me like a señora.

It was an overnight phenomenon. One day I was a naive, bright-eyed señorita y al otro día toda una mujer casada: una señora. A full-fledged woman. Suddenly, the women in my family started talking to me about Tupperware, recipes, taking care of my husband, waking up to make him breakfast, and pack his lunch for work, and that I needed to get the biggest size of Fabuloso cleaner para que me dure más. First of all, lavender Fabuloso all the way. Second of all, our kitchen was so small I needed like two drops of Fabuloso para trapear the whole thing. Third of all, what the fuck is happening!? Did I marry a child that can't do any of these things on his own? Why do I have to do all of that? Will he leave me if I don't clean?

My mom and Tita came to visit us in Seattle about two months after the wedding. I was excited to show them my new city. So, we woke up early to make the most of the day.

"¿Listas? ¡Vámonos!" I said.

They looked at me como si hubiera matado a alguien. "¡¿Cómo que nomás así te vas a ir?! ¿Ya le preparaste el desayuno a tu marido? ¿Qué se va a llevar de lonche? Nos tenemos que esperar a que se despierte para que te despidas. Ni se te ocurra despertarlo al pobrecito."

"Ha!" I laughed and said, "He knows how to cook, and he also knows how to buy food for himself. ¡Vámonos!"

They left feeling as guilty as little girls sneaking out of the house. I could tell they were both ashamed, like they didn't raise me right, yet proud that I had the independence to not revolve around a man.

The expectation that a marriage is equivalent to a woman serving a man is dangerous. Historically, most women have gone into marriage knowing they'd be essentially caregiving for their husband for the rest of their lives. It is dangerous because men also are raised believing that women are meant to be their servants and, if they don't obey, they are asking to be hit, yelled at, or discarded. This isn't love: it is a threat. As an ex-wife who received shame and blame while everyone called my ex-husband a pobrecito, it is infuriating. The unspoken rule is: if you obey and submit and clean and take care of me, I won't have to control you, yell at you, hit you, or humiliate you into being a good woman. Pero si no, pobrecita de ti, mujer. This postulates marriage as a toxic transaction rather than a loving and equitable commitment. It is an abusive relationship in which a man is treating his wife like a possession and object. This is not love. In order for the secondary order of change to occur, we need to stop calling abuse and codependency love. We need to redefine love for ourselves and begin by loving ourselves.

From a young age we were taught to control and be controlled by men; to possess and be possessed. "He is the head, you are the neck," they said. I think at one point I even believed it was in the Bible.

Codependence has the power to consume your life and spit it back out and leave you to clean up the mess. It has you constantly giving to others while emptying yourself. We become shells of ourselves, sometimes to the point that we forget who we truly are. We see women expertly caring for everyone, yet they have no idea how to care for themselves. People pleasers, martyrs, clingers, and those who are withering excuses of who they used to be—codependents go by many names and take on various roles. If you ask a codependent how others are doing, they can tell you what everyone else is feeling, what they need, and how they may respond. If you ask them what they need and how they are feeling, you may get a look of utter confusion and shock as if what they need never occurred to them. Codependents often find themselves in chaotic situations with chaotic people and will try to control the chaos yet feel completely overwhelmed and stretched thin. We empty ourselves and then blame other people for it. We often care too much, and we become obsessed with people who care too little.

Codependent relationships often feel like we are pouring in love, time, energy into an empty bucket. It feels like a bottomless pit we give everything to and get nothing back in return. Yet we stay, and we tolerate, and we give, and we love and we nurture and we become less and less ourselves while giving more and more to everyone else. We stop living our own lives and become consumed with everyone else's.

It gets to the point where you have to make a conscious choice to live your life. You have to choose to become responsible for you again. You need to reclaim your power and agency to heal and recover. These obsessive behaviors sometimes gave us a sense of control. Other times we used it as an attempt to fill the empty spaces or distract ourselves from our own needs and pain. We use other people's problems to distract us from our own. At times, we don't know how to get out even when it becomes unhealthy and unsafe.

We feel powerless when it comes to love. Soon we are so involved in other people's lives that our own lives become unmanageable. We start taking care of everyone and leave ourselves last. All of this in the name of love. Wounded love. Mujer, we want a love that gives us wings—an expansive love, not an expensive love that costs us everything, including our soul.

Codependency can be a life-threatening condition in so many ways, and our cultura creates ripe conditions for it. We see so many of our mothers, tías, and abuelas living their lives for everyone else. They forget what they like, their dreams, or how to do things for themselves. Their lives are so cluttered with everyone else's needs they forget they have needs themselves. Melody Beattie, one of the leading experts on codependence, defines codependence as the following: a person who has let another person's behavior affect him or her, and who is obsessed with controlling that person's behavior. She describes two common denominators: being in relationships with needy, troubled, or dependent people, and the set of silent yet deadly rules these relationships tend to abide by. Some of these rules include unhealthy or inexistent discussions about problems, prohibiting open and honest expression of feelings; unrealistic expectations, the inability to trust others; and no fun or play, all of which inhibit one's sense of freedom. These rules, patterns, and behaviors can become self-destructive and make the person's life unmanageable. Beattie shares that some experts say "codependents want and need sick people around them to be happy in an unhealthy way" which may seem harsh and counterintuitive.[2] However, if there is a wound and core belief—that we don't deserve happy, healthy, amor del bonito—then it is understandable we seek relationships which will keep us unhappy, unhealthy, y sufriendo, because it is familiar and because it is what we believe we deserve. Pero, mujer, you have suffered enough.

Say it with me: "I have suffered enough."

Codependency leads us to surround ourselves with self-destructive people who, in turn, destroy us and/or teach us to destroy ourselves. Codependence enters our lives like a disease which robs us of everything—especially our peace of mind. Recovery from codependence teaches us we can only control one person: us. Ourselves only. We tend to adopt these codependent tendencies because it was expected of women. We were taught that submission, caregiving, and enduring mistreatment were all desirable feminine attributes. These traits were indoctrinated to many as the ideal woman or marriage material. She will take care of you, put up with you, and never leave you. The women we saw in our lives were praised for their selflessness: lack of self. They were not full of themselves, because they were full of everyone else. They were empty of themselves: not knowing who they were, what they need, and much less what they wanted. They learned to want what their husband wanted. They learned not to need anything. They were what everyone else wanted them to be.

Codependency can be broken up into the following traits and characteristics: Caretaking, Low Self-esteem, Obsession, Controlling, Denial, Dependency, Poor Communication, Weak Boundaries, and Lack of Trust. Inspired by Beattie's *Codependent No More: How to Stop Controlling Others and Start Caring for Yourself* [3], approach the following exercise as an opportunity to reflect on the way you or the women around you are. If you recognize the patterns below, draw a check mark next to them:

I feel:

— Responsible for taking care of other people

— Anxiety and guilt when other people have problems

— Compelled to help others solve their problems

— Like I don't know why others don't do the same for me

— Sad, like I spend my whole life giving and not receiving the same in return

— Like my wants and needs are not important

— Restless when I don't have drama in my life

— Like I overcommit myself

— Underappreciated, taken advantage of, or used

— Afraid of rejection

— Like I'm different from everyone else and I don't belong anywhere

— Like I'm not good enough

— Guilty when I do things for myself

— Uncomfortable when I receive compliments or praise

— Stupid and I beat myself up when I make a mistake

— Ashamed of who I am

— Like I have to apologize for everything

— That I don't deserve good things, new opportunities, or happiness

— Like my purpose in life is reliant on other people

— Like I can't be myself

— Like I have to prove myself to people constantly

— Like I have trouble being spontaneous and living in the moment

— Like I need to know everything that will happen before making a decision

— Like I can't trust other people because I don't trust what they'll do

— Like staying busy is what makes me feel valued

— Anxious when thinking about other people's problems, feelings, and opinions

— Like I can't stick to a routine because something always comes up

— Like my life is always overwhelming

— Like I will never be loved by romantic partners, friends, or my parents

— Like I lose myself in relationships

— Anxious when talking about myself

— Like I can never stand up/defend myself

Remember, the number of statements and sentiments that resonate with you or remind you of your family members is not meant to feel shameful. In fact, your awareness of them should be celebrated—once they are brought to light, you can begin to uproot the causes and heal them. With awareness, we can bring medicine: healing and recovery.

Although people who struggle with codependency may try to keep it all together, we see clearly that they do not. If this is you, you may find yourself helping everyone around you but yourself. You may feel helpless and unable to see how to untangle yourself from another person or group of people. One of the most important steps in recovering from codependency is detaching yourself from the people, places, and things which have consumed your time, energy, and essence. Detachment means releasing control of things outside of you and staying in touch with yourself. Pour your love and energy into yourself. Focus on yourself. Treat yourself with the same kindness, care, and concern that you invested in other people. Examine what (and who) you've been holding on so tightly to. Many times, we let go of ourselves so we can cling to someone else. Visualize and then practice actually letting them go.

Detachment doesn't mean a hostile or sudden cutoff. You can detach with love—for yourself and for them. Boundaries are essential in this process. Detachment gives back to each person the responsibility for themselves. I am responsible for me, and you are responsible for you. I will stop trying to solve your problems, control you, and do things for you that you can do for yourself. I cannot change you or fix you. I cannot speak for you or have you speak for me. I will respect your time, needs, and wants, knowing that they are your own and that they are different than mine. I will return to you the freedom to grow, learn, and be yourself, and by doing this, I return the same freedom to myself. This is loving. This is setting oneself free. It is healing.

Lo bonito es que hay medicina y sanación. We can stop abandoning ourselves and return to ourselves. We can take back our power and embrace ourselves. No se tiene que seguir viviendo así. We can learn to love ourselves and pick up the pieces of ourselves we've left behind and neglected. You can learn to feel your feelings, listen to your own voice, make decisions for yourself, think your own thoughts, set your own schedule, pursue your goals, value your opinions, and give yourself a new chance at life. Sí se puede. Trust. Confía.

> We learned to abandon ourselves by watching our mamis and abuelas abandon themselves. We were raised to sacrifice ourselves and put others first. We were raised to put el qué dirán on a pedestal, to please everyone and receive shame when we please ourselves. Yet there comes a point in every woman's life in which she feels her fire fading. There is a whisper desde las profundidades de su alma que dice: "Me estoy muriendo." We are faced with a choice, a fork in the road: "Rescue yourself or continue to sacrifice, to give of yourself until there is nothing left." El fuego se está apagando. ¿Lo vas a encender de nuevo o vas a dejarlo morir?
>
> Mujer, don't abandon yourself.
>
> Love yourself.
>
> Lucha por ti.
>
> Agárrate desde el alma y no te dejes ir.
>
> Fan your fire into a flame.
>
> Tienes todo lo que necesitas.

Break the cycle of self-abandonment. Be a woman who chose herself. Be a woman who is committed to herself. Una mujer que luchó por sí misma y ganó.

You either spend the rest of your life learning to love yourself or grieving the parts of you that are dying while you're still alive.

Es tu decisión.

Tú vales la pena.

Tu vida y tu voz valen la pena.

Your needs and your wants are worth it.

You are worth it, mujer.

No te dejes.

No te abandones.

Lucha por ti,

y gana.

Throughout my life, I had to find other women to take me under their wings and teach me. Most of these women were writers and artists who dared to say things no one was saying. They lived and loved differently. I see them as my chosen madrinas. bell hooks is one of those women. Hers is one of my favorite definitions of love. In her book *All About Love*, she writes, "Love is the will to extend one's self for the purpose of nurturing one's own or another's spiritual growth. Love is as love does. Love is an act of will—namely, both an intention and an action . . . never simply a feeling."[4] Growing up, I was taught love is a feeling, and now I realize it is so much more. It is a revolution that starts with me, and yours starts within you.

Que Viva el Amor

One of the most damaging lies passed down across cultures and generations is that love and marriage should only be between a man and a woman. This has caused too many unnecessary deaths, hate crimes, suicides, and repressed lives. It is heartbreaking. The homophobic messages we receive about love plant seeds of self-hatred and fear in those of us with queer little hearts. I grew up being afraid of loving and being loved partly because I was told I couldn't love who I wanted to love—myself included.

This message is rooted in the systemic homophobia brought forth by colonization. It has brought more heartbreak than love. Colonizers would forcibly convert indigenous peoples to their religion. They brought shame, rape, diseases, and fear. Condemning people for loving someone outside of a heterosexual relationship does not feel very loving. It is oppressive, dangerous, and mean. Too many men and women were robbed of the opportunity to experience love as they deserved due to homophobia and heteronormativity. To this day, I wish I grew up knowing I had the option to love and be loved by a woman. My life and relationships would have looked entirely different. I grieve the years I spent in the closet pretending to love men. I grieve for the men and women who never got to come out of the closet and love who they wanted to love. Love is for every-body. Love is a genderless, powerful energy that should be fully accessible to everyone, everywhere. Todos merecemos amor sin juicio y sin temor. Ni el matrimonio ni mucho menos el amor le pertenece solo a los heterosexuales. The heterosexuals shouldn't be the only ones with free access to marriage and love.

May this generation of queers grow up knowing we may love and marry whoever we choose—without shame or self-hate. I hope the next generations know queer love is beautiful and something worthy of being celebrated. I pray the next generation of queer beings grow up loving themselves. May queer folks everywhere take off the weight of the shame and blame. May we dress ourselves with shameless, revolutionary love.

Reflexiones

Write a letter of commitment to yourself. Let your mind flow, using these prompts as a loose guide. Don't overthink. Just write. Once you are done, read it out loud.

- *Perdóname por abandonarte.*

- *De estas maneras:*

- *Con estas personas:*

- *Ahora sé que lo hice porque:*

- *Now I know that you deserve better.*

- *I commit to never abandoning you again.*

- *You deserve a type of love that…*

- *I will make sure you give yourself this love by…*

- *Mujer, te amo y siempre te amaré.*

Abrázate y nunca más te sueltes, mujer.

ABUSE

"¿Qué va a decir la gente?"

"Así son los hombres."

Abuse is one of the least talked about things in our culture, yet one of the most prevalent. It thrives on our silence. It survives in the dark. Abuse loves secrecy, and our families raised us to be quiet: Lo que pasa en la familia, se queda en la familia. The values of familismo. We must protect the family at all cost. When abuse happens within family members or to a family member it is common in our culture to refuse to talk about it, not hold the abuser accountable, and simply try to cover it up and move on as if nothing ever happened.

I was more scared to speak up about the abuse than of the abuse itself. Somehow, I knew my consequences would be harsher if I spoke up, rather than my abuser. It took me years to gather the courage to say anything. My family responded in punishing ways, which made me question my decision to speak—and myself. I was breaking the number-one rule: Lo que pasa en la familia, se queda en la familia. They said I was ruining the family. My voice, my truth, a mujer speaking up about the abuse, was ruining the family. Not one of the adults I told blamed the abuser. Our family system was so deeply rooted in machismo that when a woman spoke up the whole system felt threatened and proceeded to silence the woman rather than hold the abuser accountable.

The ones who attacked me the most after I broke the silence were the women in my family. They said I was playing the victim and seeking attention. They said I was weak. "Stop feeling sorry for yourself and get over it." The older women in my family told me about all the abuse they had had to aguantar. They even said it with a hint of pride as they looked down upon me—like I was less of a woman for not tolerating the abuse. According to them, I was weak for not staying calladita. They accused me of victimizing myself when I spoke up and held my abuser accountable. No one asked me how I was feeling or what I needed to heal.

In the larger forest of our families, unspoken abuse is a disease. Thriving on silence, it spreads from one person to the next, from the abusers to the enablers to the survivors. Some of us only realize later in life that what has happened to us is abuse. Some of us have witnessed it and have carried the weight of emotions associated with it. An abuser can be anyone, from our parents, extended family members, siblings, partners, friends, or any number of other people in our lives. Its prevalence in our community makes it our responsibility to recognize it.

There are many different types of abuse. We will focus on the seven most prominent. Learning to identify abuse as abuse can sometimes be the first thing someone needs to remove themselves or someone they love from an abusive person and/or situation.

Physical Abuse
When a person causes physical harm to another by:
- Hitting, slapping, punching, kicking, burning, strangulation, damaging personal property, refusing others medical care, controlling medication, coercing partner into substance abuse, use of weapons

Emotional Abuse
When a person seeks to control another through:
- Name-calling, insulting, blaming, extreme jealousy, shaming, humiliation, intimidation, isolation, stalking

Sexual Abuse

When a person seeks power over another though sexual behavior performed without consent, such as:

- Forcing someone to have sex with other people, any sexual activity during which the victim is not fully conscious or cannot/is afraid of saying no, hurting a partner physically during sex, forcing a partner to have sex without protection

Technological Abuse

Using technology to control, stalk, or harm another by:

- Hacking, using tracking devices, monitoring online activity, demanding access to partner's private information

Financial Abuse

Using money to maintain power and control over another by:

- Inflicting physical harm or restraining a person from being able to attend work, harassing a partner in their workplace, controlling money and access to money, damaging a person's credit score

Spiritual Abuse

Using religious power or beliefs to shame and control people by:

- Preventing someone from practicing their religious beliefs, forcing their religious beliefs on someone else, using a person's beliefs to manipulate or shame others, forcing children to be raised in a faith that the partner has not agreed to, using religious texts or beliefs to minimize or rationalize abusive behaviors (physical, financial, emotional, or sexual abuse/marital rape)

Abuse by Immigration Status

Threatening to use or expose a person's immigration status to harm or maintain power and control over them by:

- Destroying their immigration papers, restricting the person from learning English, threatening deportation, threatening to hurt the person's family in their home country.*

The deep-rooted commitment to silencing abuse in order to protect the family poses a danger to our communities. Mexico is at the top of the list when it comes to cases of child and adolescent abuse. There are about 5.5 million cases of childhood abuse reported each year.[5] In about 30 percent of the cases reported, the abuser was the stepdad, and in 40 percent they were boys and men living within the household, or close friends of the family. A vast majority of the time, these cases went unreported, and when they were reported about 90 percent resulted in the perpetrator being released with no consequences.[6] This cultivates a sense of collective hopelessness within the system and within our homes.

One of my clients shared the sense of betrayal she felt after disclosing abuse by her stepbrother to her mother. She recalls her mom telling her, "No creo que él te haya hecho eso. No digas nada, porque no queremos más problemas en la familia." There is a sense of betrayal because our mothers and our cultura have chosen to protect perpetrators rather than uprooting a problematic system. It can inflame the additional wounds we are trying to heal, such as our

---

*   Important notice: Undocumented immigrants have certain rights and protections in the United States, and there are agencies and hotlines that offer legal, medical, and housing resources for undocumented immigrants (thehotline.org and NNIRR.org).

madre wounds, when the people we hope will support us in fact turn against us. We cannot continue blaming the victims for speaking up. Se enojan cuando no nos callamos. Us using our voice prevents them from continuing to ignore the problem. You using your voice demands they listen to something they don't want to hear: "There is an abuser in the home. I am hurting. Do something. Help me. Protect me. Stop looking away." You are not the problem. The abusers are the problem. The system rooted in machismo and toxic familismo is the problem. You weren't and aren't the one to blame. The shame was never meant for you to carry, mujer. The shame belongs to the one who should be ashamed: the abuser, not the abused. The only thing you need to be holding is yourself, con amor y cariño.

It took me years to process this. It took me years to internalize and relearn love. I had to redefine what love was and felt like to me. I had to extract abuse from my definition of love. I want a way of loving and being loved in which abuse is not part of the equation. I want a regulated nervous system in the people I love, among whom feeling at ease and safe is the highest priority. Extricating myself from relationships (including my family system) in which abusive behaviors were tolerated or perpetrated in the name of love was an act of liberation. It was me saying, "I no longer tolerate abuse in the name of love. I no longer stay in abusive situations simply because I love the person, or they claim to love me. I now have a different definition of love in which abuse isn't tolerated." I have chosen to love myself more, and this means removing myself from people and places that aren't loving toward me.

Say this with me: I am worthy of a love without abusive behaviors and patterns. I am worthy of receiving love that heals. El amor no se trata de aguantar, se trata de amar y sanar.

Reflexiones

- *What is your definition of love? What does love feel like to you?*

- *Who has loved you well in your life? What did that look and feel like? What do you need to feel loved?*

- *How are you developing healthy and loving relationships in your life? Include the relationship with yourself.*

- *What are the relationships and spaces in which you have been tolerating abusive behaviors? Are you willing and ready to remove yourself, or set loving boundaries for yourself in these situations?*

SEX

"Si regalas la leche, nadie va a querer comprar la vaca."

"De esas cosas no se habla. Eso no es de señoritas."

"A las que les gusta el sexo son putas."

"Si haces eso, Dios te va a castigar."

"La que no es virgen, es puta."

"Esas cosas son del diablo."

"No seas fácil."

In many culturas, ours included, a woman's worth is mainly determined by who she is with sexually and how many people she's been with. There's importance given to a woman's virginity. There is value attached to how many sexual partners a woman has had. This, again, is perversely attached to upholding patriarchal values set on controlling and minimizing a woman's agency, rights, body, voice, and pleasure.

Slut shaming and marianismo are very common and very harmful. We call mujeres fáciles, putas, regaladas, y descaradas. Virginity is worshiped. Sex is condemned unless it is for reproducing or under marriage as a duty to your husband. There are studies that show marianismo leads to self-silencing, which increases our risk for depression and anxiety.[7] Due to marianismo, women are expected to act like the holy mother of Jesus while men are out there running around like Satanás. Que no mamen. Bueno, que mamen y dejen mamar sin juzgar. When women aren't virgin-like, they are shamed. La que no es virgen es puta. We are told we have the Jezebel spirit. I've been called a Jezebel and whore quite a few times. By my mom. By my Tita. By angry picket-sign holders in the streets of Seattle.

Sometimes we have to be the ones to have the sex talk with our mamis, tías, o abuelas. Many of them grew up believing that sex was one of those "cosas de las que no se habla" and that sex was something secret and shameful. I believe it is something sacred and pleasurable. I also believe it isn't something to be ashamed of. It isn't only for straight people. It is beautiful. Our bodies and conchas are divine, beautiful, and worthy of pleasure and of being enjoyed. Mi abuela told me que le daba asco. It broke my heart thinking about her growing up being disgusted by her own body.

I had the sex talk with my grandmother one day over cafecito. I usually stay at mi Tita's house whenever I go to LA. Our mornings start with cafecito, galletas de animalito, y chisme. This time the vibe was off. I could feel her staring at me. She was quiet. I took a sip of my coffee and looked at her. She was giving me the stink eye. We took turns: stare, pause, sip. Until I asked her why she was looking at me all weird. She responded: "¿Tú sabes cómo tienen sexo las lesbianas?" I spit out my coffee. This was definitely not what I was expecting. I took a deep breath and said, "Sí, Tita." She gave me another stank eye before asking, "¡¿Y a ti te gusta comer concha?!" Trying my best to keep a serious face, I said, "No, Tita, no me gusta—¡ME ENCANTAAAA!" Her face filled with bewilderment. She was too shocked to speak until she gave me a gentle slap and said, "¡Cállate! ¡Cochina!" She told me how disgusting she thought vaginas and vulvas were. She said everything about them grossed her out, including her own. From her comments, it was clear no one had ever pleasured her in this way, and it was frightening for her to even think about it. We talked about how sex between two women can be completely different than heterosexual intercourse. I let her know how sacred it felt to be physically intimate with a woman. I loved having the opportunity to introduce a different narrative for her. Not only did I tell her I loved my concha, but I also loved other women's conchas preciosas. Not only did I tell her I enjoyed sex and found it beautiful, I spoke to her about queer sex. She told me I was the one and only person she'd ever talked to about this. There was something powerful for me when I realized I was having this conversation without shame. We bring revolutionary healing when we dismantle shame from our narratives, bodies, and pleasure.

Many of us grew up hearing about sex only within the context of shame. It's time for that to change. Como siempre, it starts with us.

Reflexiones

- *What are ways in which you can uproot the shame from your body, sex, and sensuality? What does planting seeds of love and liberation look like? Do you experience feelings of shame tied to sex and pleasure? When are they strongest?*

- *What did you hear, if anything, from your mamá, tías, o abuelas about sex?*

- *What are the things about sex and your body you wish you'd heard growing up? How would you give your inner niña the sex talk without shame and blame?*

WORK & MONEY

"Búscate a un hombre que te mantenga."

"Las mujeres no deben trabajar; deben quedarse en casa."

"Money comes from men and they control it."

"Estudia para que nunca tengas que depender de un cabrón."

"Hide what you spend from your man."

For those of us who grew up in poverty, it is hard to unlearn the fear and desperation that comes with scarcity. According to U.S. Census Bureau data, 17 percent of Latines lived in poverty in 2022[8]—that's roughly 10 million Latine people living without the resources they need. Sometimes growing up not having enough is internalized as not being enough. There are a lot of factors that contribute to the prevalence of poverty among our people. A lot of it is traced back to colonization and machismo.

My mom was a secret compulsive shopper. She'd go shopping and hide the evidence from her men. The first time I was in on the secret was when she bought us those double-tipped, scented markers. They had a regular marker felt tip on one end and on the other they had cool shapes like a heart, clover, moon, stars, etc. My mom told us not to say anything and not to bring them out when Oscar was home. He'd be mad we were spending his money on stupid things. Mostly because we didn't have any. Whatever money we did have belonged to him because he was the one that worked. This was a belief that permeated throughout most of the family units in my family system across generations. Men worked; women stayed home. Men earned the money; women depended on them and their money. Men made all the financial choices.

Financial dependence increases the risk for abuse and is sometimes used by perpetrators of domestic violence to hold power and control over their victims.[9] There are men who don't let their wives work in order to prevent them from gaining independence and financial agency. There is nothing wrong with this per se, if it is your personal choice. However, if we grow up believing it is our only choice, or not believing in ourselves enough to be financially independent, then it is time to start reframing some of our core beliefs around money, men, and mujeres.

Many of us were raised believing that one of our main goals in life should be to marry a rich man who could support us and our babies so that we didn't have to work. The quality of the man and the health of the relationship doesn't matter. Many women find themselves in relationships in which they are suffering silently from the moment they marry to the moment they die. For me, it felt like a slow, silent, and suffocating sacrificing of myself. My agency was fleeting. I knew that was not how I wanted to keep living. I knew my former husband had more power, privilege, and money than me. Shortly after our divorce, we went to the bank to separate our accounts. He left me with less than five hundred dollars to my name. I didn't ask for anything because I wanted the divorce to be fast and easy. I knew he would fight me if I asked for money. I would rather lose it all than keep living that life. The divorce forced me to trust myself enough to survive and thrive on my own. Más bien, I was and did better off without him.

I learned I needed to, and could, depend on myself not only financially, but in every way.

I've seen too many mujeres stay with abusive men because of money. They depended on a man to the point that they couldn't leave him and survive. It gets more complicated if there are children involved and/or if the person trying to leave is undocumented. We must consider the complexities of why it is so difficult for women to become financially stable and independent. There are many obstacles between money and mujeres. One of the biggest obstacles is men and the systemic structures built to keep men in power and with more direct access to wealth. Current immigration policies and lack of access to childcare, work qualifications, education, community support, healthcare, transportation, housing, and access to other resources are obstacles to consider when we think about women and wealth—and how they can build intergenerational wealth.

We are often taught to care for and prioritize everyone but ourselves. This also applies to money. We use most of our money to survive or take care of others. However, we are not taught how to use it to invest and take care of ourselves.

Scarcity tells us we don't have enough. Abundance tells us we are more than enough. Scarcity keeps us in survival mode. Abundance invites us to live with and build generational wealth, enjoy life without worries or guilt, and simply live without the fear of not having enough. Abundance invites peace. We want peace. It is so much more than the quantity you have in your bank account. There are a lot of people with big bank accounts, yet they do not live in abundance because their mentality is still one of scarcity. They hoard the money and, at their core, still believe they do not have enough and that it will never be enough. Mujer, you are more than enough. May your mind, love, and life be abundant. Te lo mereces.

Reflexiones

- *What does abundance look like to you? How do you want that abundance to make you feel?*

- *Think of the women in your life and their relationship to money. Can you see some of your habits reflected in them?*

- *What are the resources you need to feel financially secure?*

- *Practice inviting abundance into your life. Visualize what your life would look like if you had abundance in your finances, relationships, dreams, work, self-perception, etc. Write it down.*

- *What are the obstacles that prevented your family from obtaining intergenerational wealth? How are you going to change this?*

MENTAL HEALTH

"Yo no necesito ir a terapia porque tengo a Jesús."

"La terapia es para gringos y locos."

"Si estás aburrida o triste, ponte a limpiar."

"Si sigues llorando, te voy a dar razones para llorar."

"Yo sí tenía razones para deprimirme, tú no. Tienes todo lo que yo nunca tuve."

"Si supieras lo que yo pasé."

When I told my mother I was going to therapy she acted like I had just slapped her in the face. She got mad and told me they were going to brainwash me. "You better not talk shit about the family." This was unheard of in my family. Why would I pay to go to a stranger to tell them about our family problems?! ¡Eso no se hace! ¡Qué horror! Me choosing to go to therapy threatened our family system. Hence, the resistance. I was certain I wanted to do it and I needed to heal. Mi mami hit me with the "I don't need therapy because I have Jesus."

I hit her back with: "I respect the way you have chosen to heal. Let me know how it works for you. I also have Jesus, and just like people go to the doctor when they are sick, I am going to go to therapy because I want to heal. Jesus won't leave me for going to therapy." She made a fuchi face. I told her that I felt like I'd lived my whole life with a broken arm. It hurts. I learned to adjust and cope with doing things with one arm. Just like we go to the doctor for a broken arm, I was going to therapy for my bruised-up heart. Sometimes, the doctor has to break the arm again if the bone doesn't heal correctly. I'd rather have my arm reset and have it heal so I can use both arms, rather than spend the rest of my life with a broken arm. I want to live my life with two healthy arms and an open heart. There's just so much more we can do and be when we heal.

En mi familia, therapy was seen as a white-people thing, para locos. We were told it was not for people like us. Again, we had to uphold the silence. Going to talk to a therapist was violating that unspoken agreement to maintain the silence. Part of the fear that comes up for our families when we mention going to therapy is rooted in familismo. In centripetal family systems, which center the family, bringing in strangers or people from the outside is dangerous and a threat to the family system. This is especially true for dysfunctional and frágil systems in which silence upholds the current abusive systems in place. Usually, those with more power in the family system are the ones who demand the most silence and loyalty. However, mi Tita taught me a phrase that I'd like to apply here: el que nada debe, nada teme (the one who owes nothing, fears nothing). Many are afraid of us sharing our stories in therapy because they have played harmful or villainous roles in them.

Although the general resistance to therapy has to do with fear and shame, there's also another factor I'd like to acknowledge. One of the biggest underlying reasons my family was scared of therapy was that they were undocumented. They feared that if I spoke up about them being undocumented this could increase their chances of being deported. If I spoke about the abuse happening at home, it would also get them deported. I was afraid of this too. Although I needed to talk about this in order to heal, I didn't know who I could trust. I didn't want therapy to be the reason my mom got deported and we ended up in foster care. This was a huge weight on my shoulders. My mom would always warn us: "Si me llevan o me deportan, ¿qué les va a pasar a ustedes?"

It wasn't until I had laid everything bare and my feelings had been contained by a professional that I truly began doing some of the necessary work to heal the unprocessed trauma and shame I'd been carrying for years. I'd look forward to my therapy days. Although they were emotionally depleting, I knew that each time I'd come out a little stronger and more aware. I was actively and intentionally working on my healing. I was getting to know me. The trauma was no longer living in my body.

Therapy was where I first learned about boundaries. It was also where I learned how important culturally and trauma-informed care is. Most of my therapists were white. I had to translate and explain a lot of the cultural values, context, and nuances about my life, experiences, and family system. My mouth dropped open when my first therapist told me that my mom was a narcissist and I needed to cut her off.

"You don't owe her anything. She is toxic. You could cut her off and never talk to her again if you wanted to. She was not a good mother to you and, sadly, she never will be."

¡Vieja loca!

How dare she tell me to stop talking to my mom? At that point in my life, it felt like she was nonchalantly telling me to cut off my own leg. I couldn't fathom the idea. I told her not talking to our moms was not something us Mexicans could do. It simply was not an option for me. Now, after years of therapy and research, I understand there are situations where cutoff is necessary. I am not the biggest advocate for cutoff, but I do consider it a choice at times when it is the least harmful option.

However, back then, I almost stopped going to therapy after she told me that. My therapist would say things that made her seem like the crazy one. There would be times she'd be crying, and I had to give her the tissue. I had a hard time crying and feeling the feelings because I was still numb from all of the trauma. I had to give her the tissues and ended up feeling bad for making my therapist cry when she heard how fucked up my life had been thus far. Clearly, she hadn't grown up in the hood or had clients with complex trauma. Maybe she was having a normal human reaction and showing me what empathy looked like. Even though I would've been able to receive it better if I knew she knew more about my culture, how tough things are in the hood, and how Latine family systems work, therapy modeled empathy for me. I hadn't had much experience with empathy. It made me uncomfortable. It also helped me heal. I eventually switched therapists because I got tired of translating and explaining. I didn't want to have to educate my therapist on my experience. I wanted to be held. I wanted to be the one crying. After a few tries, I found a Latina therapist who understood and was able to hand me the tissues while I cried and processed my trauma.

Poco a poco, I could feel the therapeutic process actually working. It helped me find my voice. The trauma that once used to be stuck and buried deep in the crevices of my shame slowly began to leave my trembling body. The process was never linear. It was not pretty either. Therapy is for the brave. I'd purposely not wear make up on the days I had therapy, because I knew it wasn't about being pretty. It was about being real. After therapy, I'd grab a giant bag of hot Cheetos and drink red wine. I'd lay on the couch and cry, like real ugly crying. The type of ugly crying that scared my cat. Me entregué completamente al proceso. I surrendered fully to the process because I desperately wanted to heal. I didn't want to live with so much trauma, pain, and shame buried in my body, wrapped around me, suffocating me. The healing journey felt like a baby's first gasp for air. My first words. Reclaiming la voz de mi alma.

Therapy gave me hope to heal so that I could use both arms. It will hurt at first because the broken arm will probably have to be broken again in order to set it right, but at the end I would have two functioning arms. The things I could do with two healthy arms. I could hold myself. I could hug more people. I could dance and lift and paint. Most importantly, the wound would heal. Por fin.

I even became a licensed therapist myself. For so long, therapy has mostly been accessible to white, upper middle-class folks. We are still vastly underrepresented and have very limited access to affordable, culturally aware, trauma-informed therapy. Latine therapists represent about 5 percent of the therapists in the United States. These language and cultural barriers limit access to quality care for Latine and Spanish-speaking clients.[10] Our parents and their parents were busy surviving. Therapy didn't seem like a feasible option. It wasn't a resource anyone offered or made accessible to them. Although it shouldn't be, access to mental health resources is a privilege. I feel very honored to be one of the few queer Latine therapists. It's been healing to feel myself becoming the therapist I needed when I began going to therapy. I needed a therapist who understood my Spanglish and how Latine family systems work. It was exhausting and exasperating to have to educate and translate for therapists my experience on being a queer, Latina, first-generation woman over and over again.

Our generation is moving from surviving to learning to heal and love and fly. Our mamis and abuelas were taught that crying, vulnerability, and talking about your feelings was a sign of weakness. No dejes que te vean llorar. Las guapas se aguantan. No seas chillona. Depression and anxiety and other mental health diagnoses are scary, and often go unnamed and unspoken about. Over one-third of Latines in lower-income households report frequent anxiety and depression symptoms, and most go untreated due to lack of health insurance, low earnings, time flexibility, and immigration-related issues. We must also consider the stigma around therapy and mental health services in the Latine culture.[11] For example, taking medication is almost a sign that you don't trust God to heal you. At times, mental health disorders were attributed to a person being possessed by a demon. Many times, my mom tried to pray the depression and trauma out of us. Sometimes even in our sleep. It's common for parents to minimize our feelings or invalidate our experiences because they simply do not have the tools to talk about it. Oftentimes they lack the capacity to have healthy conversations about our mental health, because they'd have to face their own mental health issues. This can be overwhelming and terrifying.

When you are surviving, it is very difficult to take the time to explore your childhood trauma and feel the pain caused by your wounds. You simply can't if you have to get up and work under unjust conditions and your family is depending on you. Pero as we grow in our healing, we will begin to see how desperately our mamis and abuelas needed, and probably still need, to heal. Ellas también necesitan abrazar y sanar a sus niñas interiores. Perhaps no one told them. Perhaps you are the first person they've seen being intentional about their mental health, healing your inner niña, and breaking family cycles. Perhaps your wings will teach them to fly.

Afirmaciones

My wings tell my story, my voice holds my truth, my heart holds the courage to carry me through.

Mis alas cuentan mi historia, mi voz cuenta mi verdad, mi corazón lleva el valor para sostenerme.

Yo vengo de mujeres guerreras que dicen y viven el "¡Sí, se puede!"

I come from warrior women who live and believe in "Yes we can!"

I will hold myself like I am my favorite flower.

Me trataré como a mi flor favorita.

I will learn to release the people and things that no longer serve me.

Aprenderé a soltar a la gente y las cosas que no me sirven.

Me abrazaré a mí misma y no me soltaré.

I will hold myself and not let myself go.

I will choose myself over and over again—even when it's hard, uncomfortable, and unfamiliar.

Me escogeré a mí misma una y otra vez… aunque sea difícil, incómodo y desconocido.

These are some of the many messages we receive desde chiquitas. Perhaps we have even passed some of these messages on to the next generation. As we reflect on the messages that our mamis told us because their mamis told them, we see the importance of the words we weave between generations, between women, between souls. Nuestras palabras son importantes. Lo que decimos. Lo que callamos. Lo que escuchamos. Son semillas que sembramos.

¿Qué vas a dejar crecer en tu jardín?

I invite you to make a list of the seeds you are planting in your garden. May you plant semillas de amor, paciencia, healthy and honest communication, justice, accountability, advocacy, safety, and liberation.

PART II

THE CHRYSALIS

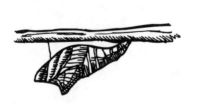

Chapter 4

The Niña Before
She Needed Healing

Inner niña work can change lives. It changed mine and I hope it will change yours. Doing this work changes our neural networks,[1] and I also believe it heals nuestros corazoncitos. There are many ways to do inner child work. For me, it is a way to honor, hear, and nurture your child self as an adult. You get to re-mother yourself y apapacharte. The word *apapachar* comes from the Nahuatl language. It means to gently caress and give love/cariño con el alma, with one's soul. Inner niña work is soul work. You bring light to the places where there was darkness. The darkness looks different for each one of us. For some, it is abuse, neglect, abandonment, numbness, grief, or unmet needs. The light is the compassion, understanding, care, cariño, and love you offer to those wounds from your past. Inner niña work can be seen as building a bridge between the shadows and the light. When we are born into trauma and suffering, it feels like growing up in the dark. We keep bumping into things, falling into the same holes, and feeling lost. This state of survival can leave our inner niñas feeling constantly scared and hopeless. Our caregivers are also surviving in this darkness and doing their best to raise us, even when they are hurting and lost themselves. People who grow up in this darkness grow up speaking a language of suffering and pain. I imagine it as if "suffering" was my first language. Como el español, we learned it first because it is the language our parents grew up speaking. As we grow up and have different life experiences, we meet other people who don't speak this language. There are people who are born into the light. Typically, these people grow up speaking a language of love and empathy. Many of us learn to speak this language poco a poquito as we grow up and begin healing. Pero we still have the accent of suffering. This also helps us recognize others who have the accent, who speak the first language. It can sometimes feel like a relief because you know that they know and you do not have to translate. This is the beauty of the bridge over which you can go to and from the light and the dark. There are times you will need to go back to the dark in order to bring light, love, and warmth, or simply sit there and feel. There are times we go back when we feel triggered. There are times we go back because it is familiar. However, as we become more familiar with this bridge between the dark and the light, we will bring light simply by being ourselves. Inner niña healing is you being the one to teach your inner child how to speak and understand love and healing as a language. It is where you get to re-mother and re-father yourself and speak those words of love and affirmation you needed to hear when you were a little girl. When you heal your inner niña you break generational cycles and plant new seeds for you to bloom and for the next generations to have more light. You are building your home in the light and bringing your inner niña with you.

At her core, your inner niña wanted to be loved, secure, heard, and held. She needed a safe adult to create a secure attachment with and develop a healthy sense of self. There are five pillars to building a secure attachment: child feels safe; child feels known (attunement); child feels comfort, soothing, and reassurance; child feels valued and delighted in; and child feels supported to explore.[2] Your inner niña needs you to be consistent, supportive, safe, soothing, present, and attuned to her. The psychological definition of attunement refers to the emotional connectedness between two people and the capacity to respond and tend to the child's needs in a consistent and effective way.[3] Many of our inner niñas did not have the attunement we needed from our parents and caregivers. We didn't feel their emotional connectedness and the consistency necessary for her to feel she can depend on us. Inner niña work is learning and leaning into this attunement process with your inner niña.

Attuning to your inner niña can look like asking her to show you which parts of her are still hurting, which parts of her need love, and which parts of her need to be held. It means teaching her how to listen to her body, mind, and corazoncito and communicating what she needs. It also means being open and capable of meeting those needs. Oftentimes, we carry unprocessed trauma in our bodies. We feel pressure in our chest, start to shake, or get an overwhelming sense of grief. There were probably times in your childhood when you experienced traumatic events and did not have the capacity to process them. When this happens, our brains and nervous systems numb, freeze, or block out the feelings and memories so they don't overwhelm us or further traumatize us. This may explain why there are certain moments in your childhood that are hard to remember, or certain emotions that are hard for you to feel.

When we experience these traumas, our emotional development tends to stop at the age when that trauma was experienced. For example, if you survived abuse or a traumatic experience at the age of nine and you didn't receive help to process the trauma, chances are your socioemotional and psychological development were impaired. You are now a woman, and within you lives the scared niña with unresolved and unprocessed trauma. She sometimes comes out when you are triggered, frightened, angry, or wounded. Your response to instability was to shut down your feelings and hide in the closet. Now, as an adult, you're with a partner and they yell at you. Your response is to shut down and hide in your car.

Part of the trauma response work we will be doing is helping you connect with that scared, traumatized niña. You will communicate with her and let her know she is safe now. You are an adult, and you will take care of her. You will not let anything bad happen to her. You will love her and protect her. She doesn't need to respond out of that wounded survival mode. You've learned and are learning new behaviors so that she doesn't have to use those old coping mechanisms. She can simply be a niña again.

According to Dr. Margarita Blanco, author of *Sanación Emocional del Niño Interior: Método Ser Mejor Ser*, we reprogram our emotional system and neurological pathways when we heal our inner child. In order to do this, we must reparent ourselves: become the mother and/or father that we needed and, frankly, still need. As we meet our inner niñas, we can learn to recognize our needs and meet them. You can connect with your inner niña in many ways: set intention and listen to her, look at old photos of you and send love, do things she loved doing, and maybe even get her the toy she always wanted but never got. The most important thing is listening to her. To do this, we need to recognize the essence of our childhood selves.

One of my clients asked me, "¿Cómo lo haces, Kim? ¿Cómo le haces cuando todo se siente tan oscuro y llegan esos pensamientos tan pesados?"

I thought about my inner niña putting all her faith in the light, even on the darkest nights. El amanecer—it still fills me with hope. One of the things I've learned to do in moments of darkness is make a list of my light sources: people, places, and things that bring me light. They are my lighthouses through the darkest, most tempestuous times. In some ways, I am like the moth who gravitates toward the light. Find your light sources and trust that you are also a source of light to many. Trust that you are a lighthouse for your inner niña to walk toward.

It's a process of remembering the version of you before you learned what fear was, before you learned what loss was, and before you knew what hurt was. There are several paths to take when reconnecting with your inner niña. Find the essence of who you are without the trauma. Many of our inner niñas were wild, outspoken, carefree, bold, creative, and imaginative before they encountered trauma. My mami always used to tell me how outspoken and sassy I was. She said I'd surprise her con lo que salía de mi boca y que nunca me callaba. I'd speak my mind and was not afraid to stand up for myself. Mi mami said I'd dance around the grocery store aisles and choreograph dances for my classmates after school. Then I encountered trauma. Fear enveloped me. I got quieter and more hypervigilant. I stopped dancing and started hiding. My light turned into a shadow.

Trauma robs us of our essence in many ways. It introduces fear, doubt, and shame. These hinder us from expanding and growing our sense of self. They obscure our ability to love ourselves and shift our self-perception. Not only do we begin to see ourselves differently when we encounter trauma or abuse, we also begin to see the world and those around us differently. We have difficulty taking up space, trusting, and feeling safe. We begin looking over our shoulder and being hypervigilant. It is hard to know who to trust and how to gauge if we are safe. Our inner niñas abandoned themselves in order to hide and survive. They stopped focusing on their development and focused on silencing and shrinking. They began centering their sense of worth on pleasing other people in order to be loved. Poco a poquito and all of a sudden, our inner niñas stopped being niñas. We became little señoras. Then, we became adults with these abandoned inner niñas still trying to survive inside us. Return your inner niña to her essence. Return that scared little niña to her joy. Return her to herself.

If you have a photo of yourself from when you were a little niña, take the time to look at her con ojos de amor. Try to remember who she was. What did the younger version of you love to do, watch, eat, listen to, etc. What were her dreams, goals, and to what did she aspire? Take time to think about the things you wanted and the things you needed back then. Take time to listen to that little corazón. Growing up we saw the mujeres in our lives also abandon themselves. Through observation or through messages they passed on, the younger versions of ourselves quickly learned that:

"I go last. My needs go last."
"I am here to serve others and sacrifice myself."
"My needs are not important."
"I am not important."
"My voice doesn't matter."
"What I want doesn't matter."
"I don't matter."

One of the most important parts about inner niña work is you actually taking the time to connect with your inner niña. It is much more than just a conceptualización of her. You must create a direct and nurturing relationship with her. Conecta con tu niña interior. This is work only you can do.

Inner Niña Visualization

One of the most intimate ways we get to connect with our inner niña is through visualization. Visualize a safe place for you to meet and invite her in. Create a place with her likes, wants, and needs in mind. Piensa en qué le gusta, qué la hace feliz, qué la hace sentir segura.

Begin by picturing this safe place. It can be a place you've been to, a beautiful place you create in your mind, or a place you've always wanted to go to. Make sure it is a place where you feel safe, free from old memories or traumas.

Picture yourself setting this space up con amor e intención. Make sure it is a place where your inner niña can walk in and know it is for her. May it be a place that centers her and is created just for her. This may be the first time she's had a space like this just for her.

Invite your inner niña to come meet you there.
Look at her con amor and simply see her.
What does she look like?
What is her essence?
What is she wearing?

Introduce yourself to her. Let her take you in. Let her see the woman she has become.
What does she see?
What does she feel looking at you?

When you feel ready, ask her to tell you about her what she likes, what is going on with her life at the time, what she needs to hear, feel, know, and see.

Listen to her.

Ask her to show you her life before the wounds and the trauma.
Ask her how she felt and what her dreams were.
Thank her for showing you. Thank her for trusting you.

Ask her to show you where she's hurting. Tell her to tell you who hurt her. What is she afraid of? Ask her to show you the darkness she's afraid of.

Ask her what she needed when she was hurting, afraid, and trying her best to be strong, and what she needs. Can you give it to her?

Give her the reassurance, apapachos, patience, compassion, and besitos that she needs.

Hold her. Abrázala fuerte y dile que ya no está sola. You have the light now. You are the light now. You've made a home in the light for her, so she does not have to fear the darkness anymore—it is no longer her home.

Tell her what she needs to hear.
Notice how she responds.

Hold her.
Love her.
Apapáchala.

Thank her for being there with you and let her know she can join you in this safe place any time.

Breathe and thank yourself for having the courage to do this work. Breathe until you feel ready to return to your present self.

If the visualization was difficult or too painful, respira. It is okay.
Es un proceso.

These are the essential questions we need to be asking ourselves and the niñas in our lives. They need to know their joy, hopes, and dreams matter. These exercises and similar ones become an act of integrating your essence, your wounds, the needs which were not met, and the things you've learned along the way.

As you do these exercises, you may get different results. Maybe you can't visualize your inner niña clearly—she appears blurry or not at all. Maybe your inner niña has nothing to say to you, or the opposite—she has plenty to say, and sometimes it's not all good. Not each visualization will have the results that we are looking for. Healing is not linear. When we approach the visualization practice, or any practice, with the goal to complete them perfectly, we are operating within the frame of perfectionism. It is an indication that we are trying to control the healing, rather than feeling it and integrating it. There are lessons to be learned in the absence of your inner niña, or her resistance to forming a relationship with you. Rather than looking at it through the eyes of loss, approach it as an opening to be the adult your inner niña needs.

Because your inner niña doesn't need another person to boss her around. She doesn't need another person to put expectations on her. What she needs is for her needs to be heard and respected. What she needs in a visualization may just be the chance to swing on the swings or play on the playground with the safety of an adult that lets her. Maybe she wants to speak freely, without someone telling her that she's being rude or loud. If your inner niña was an actual child in the room with you now, giving you the stink eye, ignoring you, or telling you like it is the way kids tend to do, you wouldn't take offense or give up on her. You would reach out and try to see how to make that child more comfortable. Be an adult and listen. Be open and witness yourself as a person that's doing the work. Apologize. Forgive. Be.

We can provide ourselves with the love, security, trust, consistency, respect, and guidance our inner child needed so desperately while we were developing our identity and making sense of our world. Once we embrace our inner niña and plant new seeds in our gardens, we will have new ways of seeing and interacting with our world. Our lives will change because our ways of viewing and holding ourselves will change. The hope is to get to a place where we will see ourselves and this world from a place of love and not from our wounds.

However painful or distant it may be, we must reconnect with the part of us from before the trauma. There is a sense of grief for who we could've been without the trauma. Guilt and shame can also be barriers keeping us from truly connecting with our inner niñas, whether it's the guilt that comes from not being able to protect her in the past, or guilt that you allowed yourself to change. You may need to ask for forgiveness and forgive your inner niña. Finding compassion for the mujer you are now and your inner niña is essential for the healing process to take root.

Por eso es importante abrazar a esa niña interior y sanarla. Those wounds were most likely inflicted by our parents or primary caregivers, who were most likely adults who were hurt, frustrated, confused, insecure, and shamed themselves. The chance that they have unhealed childhood wounds is likely. Many of our mamis and papis didn't have the privilege or time to heal their inner niños. You have the opportunity to do that now. Tienes la oportunidad de abrazar a tu niña interior y sanar.

This practice at first might be unfamiliar, especially when the world wants us to grow up so fast. The girl before the trauma may seem so far away. Almost like a figment of our imaginations. Did she even exist? What if the person we are now is very different from who we used to be? Sometimes we aren't ready to connect with our inner niña in that way. Sometimes she's not ready to connect with us. Poco a poquito. If you're struggling to find your inner niña, a veces you need to try again some other time. This is heart work and hard work. Proceed with cariño.

Ask your inner niña to show you your spark, your gifts, the magic only you can create out of nothing. It's always been within you. Dile a tu niña que te enseñe tu magia que te hace brillar. Let her grab your hand and guide you. Revisit your childhood and adolescence in search of your magic.

WHERE I COME FROM

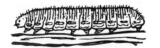

Take a moment to reflect on your roots based on all we've learned and walked through thus far. When you write about your history, roots, story, write from a place of love, understanding, cariño. Write about your inner niña and what it was like for her to grow up under those circumstances. Write in first person and don't overthink it. What was the beginning of your story like? Your childhood? What world and soil were you born into?

WHAT I INTERNALIZED
(WHAT MADE ME WHO I AM)

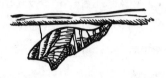

- What are the messages you received, like seeds for your garden?
- Who are the people that planted those seeds?
- What are the values and beliefs that were a part of your identity development?
- What made you, you?
- Who are the key characters in your story?
- What are the words that are still with you?
- Where are the places connected to you?
- What are the wounds, attachments, and memories that began growing in your garden?

WHAT I'VE LEARNED, UNLEARNED,
AND TRANSFORMED

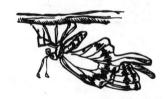

- How have you tended to your garden?
- What are the seeds you planted on your own?
- What have you made from what's grown in your garden?
- What have you transformed?
- What cycles have you broken?

- What wounds have healed, and which ones are still healing?
- How will you love yourself today?
- How will you love yourself tomorrow?
- How will you show love to who you were yesterday?

BECOMING

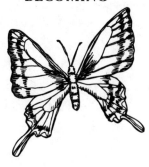

- Who are you becoming?
- How are the choices you make today informing the woman/person you become tomorrow?
- Who is the woman of your dreams?
- What changes do you need to make in your life now in order to become her?
- How would your inner niña feel if she saw her?
- Who would you become if fear, silence, and shame were not making decisions for you?

You must continue this relationship with your inner child. It is not a one-time event. It is a loving relationship in which you must learn to nurture, listen, protect, play, defend, love, y apapachar that inner niña. This inner child work is soul work. It is profound and sacred. It brings light to the darkest places and embraces the parts of you that were once abandoned. You get to remind your inner child they don't have to live in the dark anymore and that you are creating a life for them where they can heal and feel safe.

You get to provide that inner child with a new life, new home, and new way of being loved. You get to give them the life you always wanted and needed.

Take a moment to visualize your inner niña again. Hug her close and tell her:

"I am here now. I will take care of you. Yo me haré cargo de ti. You had so much on your shoulders. Eras muy chiquita para preocuparte por tanto. Ahora yo te voy a cuidar y proteger. I will take care of you and protect you now. I promise you I will be responsible for us now, so that you don't have to be. So that you can be una niña y puedas jugar y ser libre."

Tell your inner child: "The past is gone, we are in the present, and I will be with you in the future." Dile a tu niña interior: "El pasado ya pasó, estamos en el presente y estaré contigo en el futuro."

Afirmaciones

It is never too late to heal.
Nunca es demasiado tarde para sanar.

I will give the next generation what my inner niña and mi mami's inner niña needed. Soft love will be my legacy.
Le voy a dar a la siguiente generación lo que mi niña interior y la niña interior de mi mami necesitaban.
Un amor tierno será mi legado.

Sweet soul of mine, I am fighting for you.
Alma mía, estoy luchando por ti.

Chapter 5

Trauma Encounters

The first time I went to therapy was in Seattle. It was a require-
ment for my graduate school program. I was shaking from
nerves in the waiting room. When she let me into her office, the first
thing I noticed was the painting on the wall. It was a woman with a
butterfly coming out of her mouth. *I want to be like her*, I thought.
I shared my story and watched as she cried. The more I shared, the
more my body shook. It reminded me of when I was a little girl. My
family was in a four-vehicle collision when I was eight years old.
The airbag burst in my face and knocked me unconscious. I woke
up in a random lady's arms, wearing a random man's sweater, shak-
ing from the shock. From then on, whenever stressful or frightening
things would happen in my life, my body would shake and I would
go numb. I wouldn't be able to feel anything. So, as this therapist
sat there crying, I handed her a tissue and didn't feel a thing other
than the shaking in my body. The story I was telling her felt like it
belonged to someone else. When the session ended, I asked her if she

had a diagnosis for me. She looked at me as if it was obvious, "You have PTSD."

Dumbfounded, I asked, "What is that?"

"Post-Traumatic Stress Disorder. It's what some soldiers experience after a war."

On the bus ride home, I looked up PTSD. So much of what I read applied to me. It was also a bit of a shock to come to terms with the trauma I'd encountered and the impact it had on how I perceived myself and the world around me.

The trauma we encounter throughout our lives forms a part of us, one way or another. It weaves itself into our stories, worldview, and sense of self. Many of us encountered trauma, abuse, or emotional harm during our childhood and/or adolescence. How our family and primary caregivers responded to trauma and abuse plays an important role in our developmental and psychological well-being. If a child doesn't receive help and protection when they go to a trusted adult, this creates cognitive dissonance, which is transformed into internalized shame, low self-esteem, a sense of worthlessness, and learned helplessness.

These trauma encounters, or moments of heightened unsafety, can leave us feeling like there is something wrong with us, or as if we are somehow at fault. The result can sometimes be deep shame, as if it reflects who we are and not of who is abusing us. I am here to tell you: No es tu culpa. It doesn't make you any less lovable. It does not determine your worth. It does not define you. A veces estas palabras no son suficientes para quitar el dolor, la pena, las sombras de encima. El trauma entierra sus garras en lo más profundo de nuestras almas. It begins dictating our sense of self and our worldview. At times, trauma feels like a weighted blanket we can't take off. Other times, it feels like chains we don't have keys to. Many times, el trauma se siente como una mano sobre nuestra boca que nos roba el aire y no nos deja hablar. Sofocante. Suffocating.

The CDC defines trauma as an event or series of events which cause deep stress, a sense of horror, helplessness, injury, or threat of death.[1] When we look at trauma so clinically, it's easy to feel removed from it—to see it de lejitos. Oftentimes, people associate trauma with a large-scale, single event with rippling impact, but trauma can occur repeatedly and less visibly. There may be circumstances in your life that may not have felt like trauma as they were happening, but later on, you realized the impact that they had. The effects of trauma are serious. They infiltrate deep in our being, our sense of safety, and our ability to function. If they are left untreated, we carry the weight of trauma in our psyche, body, and soul. This is why it is important for us to tend to it.

Trauma, though not one-size-fits-all, is often put into three categories: acute, chronic, and complex.

> *Acute trauma* results from a single incident. This can look like a car accident, a natural disaster, or a loved one's death. Es algo que pasa de repente, una vez, but it leaves a deep impact on your life and sense of safety.
>
> *Chronic trauma* is repeated and prolonged events like abuse, domestic violence, lack of resources, neglect, harassment, illnesses, etc.
>
> *Complex trauma* is exposure to multiple and diverse traumatic encounters that are more commonly invasive to one's boundaries and safety and is interpersonal in nature.

Traumatic encounters can leave one feeling as if their sense of safety is threatened. When a child feels they are no longer safe in the world, it is a dangerous thing. Feeling unsafe during your developmental years alters your psychosocial development, as we learned when exploring ACE scores. Sadly, if we pay close enough attention, we can see which children grew up with and without trauma.[2] According to the ACE study, the children who've experienced adversity express anxiety, hypervigilance, depression, and other behavioral externalizations of their lack of safety (whether it be physical or emotional).[3] Not only is an encounter with trauma influential to a child's development, but their caregivers' response to the child's encounters are also essential determining factors for how a child processes and heals from the trauma.

What can feel traumatic for you can feel completely different to your tía. The difference in the lessons you were taught growing up, your personalities, mental health, and specific experiences can lead to completely separate perspectives about what can and can't be considered traumatic. Sometimes, the people that do not see what you've gone through as trauma have trouble reconciling that their similar encounter may also be trauma because repressing their feelings can be a survival technique. Even the places your body stores trauma or the way it goes about processing it can be different. This does not take away from either of your experiences. It is just how trauma works and how our minds and bodies respond to it. It helps to understand the types of trauma. Most importantly, it helps to understand yourself.

For my family, trauma looked like poverty: having the electricity cut off, not having enough money for well-balanced meals (often, my mom would feed all four of us with two Cup Noodles), and facing chronic housing instability. The lady that would come knock on our door, yelling and cussing my mother out, was also a source of trauma. The verbally and physically violent fights between my mother and her partners—traumatic. There were times I didn't know if there would be blood, bruises, or worse.

We weren't given the words for some of these traumatic encounters—it was just our life, and we were just surviving. It was only felt or seen. Son las cositas que nos aceleran el corazón, make us feel unsafe, our bodies tense up, que nuestro corazón se apachurre y que nos lastiman a nosotros o a nuestros seres queridos. Esto se acumula y si no se sana se guarda como trauma en nuestros cuerpos, mentes, y espíritus. Addressing your trauma can sometimes feel terrifying. It feels like you are about to dive off a cliff and into a roaring ocean. Respira. Remember you know how to swim. You will not drown in your trauma. We are doing this work so you don't belly flop into the ocean. We will take this un pasito a la vez. You can start by listening to yourself. Many of us have been too busy surviving to stop and listen. Ellen Bass and Laura Davis, authors of *The Courage to Heal*, wrote, "we cannot heal until we acknowledge the impact."[4] Part of this process requires us to slow down in order to notice and heal our wounds.

Trauma and abuse have the power to impact our self-esteem, feelings, and body, as well as our capacity for intimacy, parenting, and forming healthy relationships. When our bodies and brains experience or perceive the threat of danger or trauma, they prepare themselves to fight or flee. This moment of activation is what is usually referred to as "feeling triggered." Your system undergoes a physiological reaction that prepares you for action: your heart, blood pressure, and breath accelerate, and your body is in hypervigilance. Another possible reaction to trauma and triggers is freezing or dissociating.[5] Dissociation is a disconnection between the self, body, and surrounding environments when a person is feeling overwhelmed, severely stressed, or is experiencing traumatic or triggering situations. It is important for you to slow down and recognize what your triggers are. What are the people, places, and things that cause your system to perceive danger or remember a traumatic memory? Are you able to regulate your system and feel safe afterward? When trauma survivors do not receive the care they need following traumatic events, they cease to feel safe and often experience an acute stress reaction that may develop into PTSD.[6] Some of the most telling symptoms of those with PTSD include flashbacks, nightmares, difficulty sleeping, numbness, challenges concentrating, depression, intrusive thoughts, rage explosions, hypervigilance, heightened startle reflex, and isolation.[7] It can feel overwhelming at first to listen to your body and mind, especially after trauma has caused you to disconnect and dissociate from those feelings. However, these are waters we must navigate in order to heal. In order to not drown, we must learn how to self-soothe and practice caring for ourselves.

Self-soothing is a key to regulating your nervous system and reestablishing a sense of safety within yourself. It is learning to find your peace, even in the midst of the storm. Some people do this by breathing, visualizing or using guided imagery, praying, practicing somatic work, medication, or simply by speaking kindly to themselves. When you self-soothe, you form new neural pathways in your cerebral cortex and you slowly begin to minimize the stress responses and other PTSD symptoms.[8] Forming these new neural pathways allows your brain to understand that the abuse and trauma happened in the past and that you are creating a life in which you feel safe and loved. You are planting new seeds in your garden. You are the author of your story, mujer. You get to write a beautiful story for yourself. Your past trauma, abuse, and pain do not hold the pen to your story and truth. You do.

How the truth in our stories was received is important to how we heal. If the truth in your voice is received with empathy and honor, your own voice becomes medicine being rubbed on your wounds. Those who respond with love and compassion to your pain are part of your medicine and healing. If your truth is rejected, in a way, an essential part of you is also rejected. There is great power in your voice. However, you may not know it if people try to silence you when you're first learning to use it.

If your caregivers or trusted adults responded to your trauma in a dismissive or accusatory way, it may have caused more harm than the original trauma. How we are embraced or pushed away after our trauma disclosure plays an essential role in our healing. Most of my clients who have experienced trauma and/or abuse often tell me how their family didn't validate or hold them the way that they needed. They often felt invalidated and gaslit into getting over it and not speaking about it again. These responses usually came from caregivers in centripetal family systems who were preoccupied with "el qué dirán," keeping the family unity, and were so accustomed to trauma that they didn't see it as anything that was worth disturbing the family "peace" over. These clients usually came from families with intergenerational trauma, and many of their caregivers treated trauma as another family member. Most of these caregivers had unprocessed trauma themselves, which was usually dismissed by their own caregivers. They did not have the tools or capacity to hold my clients' trauma narrative, so they claimed to not believe it and demanded it be swept under the rug. They said, "Mejor ponte a limpiar y ya no pienses en eso." Most of them didn't know that asking you to bury your trauma next to theirs would only aggregate to your pain.

As we've explored in previous chapters, the roots and soil we were born into may not have given our caregivers the tools to embrace a traumatized niña. There are times people respond to trauma disclosure with anger, blame, silence, or by villainizing the recipient of the abuse while protecting the abuser. These harmful responses to our trauma, especially during our developmental years, plant seeds of rejection, abandonment, insecurity, silencing, and shame. As adults, we not only have to tend to the wounds and roots of trauma, but also to the wounds and roots of the way knowledge of our trauma was received. We simply got shame, rejection, and secondary trauma from those we trusted. This could sound like:

"De esas cosas no se habla."
We don't talk about such things.
"¿Qué traías puesto?"
What were you wearing?
"De seguro hiciste algo para que hiciera eso."
You must've surely done something for them to do that to you.
"Pues ya sabes cómo son los hombres."
You know how men are. Boys will be boys.
"No digas nada, porque ¿qué va a pensar la gente?"
Don't say anything, because what are people going to think?
"No te hagas la víctima. Ya pasó. Sigue adelante. Ya no pienses en eso."
Don't make yourself the victim. It happened already. Don't think about it anymore and move on.
"A mí también me pasó eso. Ni modo. Estas son las cosas que tenemos que aguantar como mujeres."
That happened to me too. Oh well, these are the things we have to put up with as women.

A healthy and loving response would involve acceptance, protection, and empathy. Your trusted person would hold and celebrate your act of courage. They would protect you and your path toward liberation. There would be action taken to ensure your physical and emotional well-being and safety. You would be provided resources and tools to heal, such as individual and family therapy, support groups with other children, and/or ancestral medicinal practices to help your spirit in its healing journey. The most important responses are the ones in which your needs are prioritized and tended to in a prompt, skilled, and loving way—without shame, blame, or an attempt to defend the abuser.

Being born into trauma or growing up with trauma is like growing up in the dark. You trip over the same things. You fall into the same holes. You can't see the way out. This is your normal. You survive. Or at least you try. The language you speak in the dark is based on suffering and survival. Fear conjugates the words you learn. When you meet someone else who speaks this language of suffering, you know they know, and no translation is needed. There is a certain camaraderie, and often an unspoken understanding.

The light and the dark are both equally important. The darkness is not necessarily bad, nor should it be demonized. I like to see my healing journey as a bridge between my light and my darkness. One is the place I was born into, and the other is the place I chose to build my home in. However, there are days I must visit the dark to bring light, medicine, and healing if it is needed. Sometimes, I visit just to remember. It is important not to forget. There are things that only the darkness could have taught me. Those lessons, experiences, and stories are worth more than gold.

When we first move into the light, we may feel like we don't belong—a little out of place. It feels like moving out of the 'hood and into a gated community with the bougie people who have never stepped foot in the 'hood. It's uncomfortable because it is unfamiliar. There is peace. You don't have to keep looking over your shoulders. Your body and mind finally have the space and safety to heal and process. You don't have to worry about surviving all the time. You get to learn to start living. Then, once you learn to live, you learn to heal. Once you learn to heal, you learn to love. Once you learn to love, you learn to enjoy your life.

There comes a moment when the light gets in. It could be through other people, therapy, love, or simply moving to a different environment. Initially, it hurts your eyes, and you shield yourself from it. It is an unknown. Slowly, your eyes become accustomed. You begin to see. You see the things you used to trip over, and you stop tripping. You see the holes and go the other way. You see the blood on your hands and on the walls. You see the way out. You see this way of living isn't the only way of living. You decide you no longer want to live in the dark. You begin letting more and more light in. Or better yet, you move out of the dark and into the light.

Your pain is valid and the healing process from trauma takes time. It is not something you can just get over or sweep under the rug. You do not have to be a victim or a villain. You were a human whose rights, boundaries, safety, and/or body were violated. This is not something that was your fault nor something that was or ever will be acceptable. No es algo que tú, ni tu mami, ni nadie tenga que volver a aguantar nunca más.

GASLIGHTING

Gaslighting is a form of emotional manipulation with the purpose of making you doubt your truth, reality, and feelings. People gaslight in an attempt to control the narrative, protect their image, and/or avoid accountability. Because this is so common, especially in emotionally abusive situations or harmful power dynamics, we normalize it and even gaslight ourselves.

Some say gaslighting often leaves you feeling defensive, confused, frustrated, and invalidated. Se siente como que no tienes una base sólida. After engaging in a conversation in which gaslighting is involved, you're often left feeling norteada, or lost—even in your own truth and experience of reality. This can be very disorienting and harmful, especially if it's a pattern or constant occurrence.

Symptoms of gaslighting include:

- You doubt yourself
- You feel like you're going crazy
- You do not trust your own opinions and decisions
- You ask everyone for permission to do anything and apologize for everything
- You fear you've done something wrong
- You feel like no one understands you or understands what you are saying

Now, imagine feeling this way desde chiquita. Many of us have felt invalidated and unheard for most of our lives. We've been purposefully silenced and taught to silence ourselves. We've been villainized when we speak up and share our emotions. Duele más when it is connected to speaking up about deep wounds and intimate details of abuse and harassment. Oftentimes we were gaslit by our caregivers, or we found partners who gaslit us because it felt familiar. By that point, we are experts at gaslighting ourselves and agreeing with those gaslighting us. Oftentimes, those who are supposed to love us the most are the ones who harm us the most. We grow up with a distorted version of what love is. It is what we know and have become accustomed to. We begin to treat ourselves the same way those who gaslight and abuse us do.

Gaslighters often dismiss you when you share your feelings, experiences, or opinions. They treat them as if they are invalid, crazy, wrong, or unimportant. If you bring up something they did or confront them on something they said, gaslighters will resort to denial tactics. It is nearly impossible for them to take accountability or admit to wrongdoing. Gaslighters will go as far as trying to convince you of false truths by forceful insistence, repetition, or fabrication of evidence to prove they are right and you are wrong. Attempting to contradict or confront a gaslighter will often result in the gaslighter questioning you and/or accusing you. When we are constantly questioned or put in positions in which we have to defend our truth, opinion, experiences, and feelings, we begin to doubt ourselves, lose an accurate perception of our own reality, and become disconnected from our own voice and needs. Isolation is a secondary byproduct of emotionally abusive situations.

Teresa, one of my therapy clients, had a very distorted sense of reality because she'd been severely gaslit by her mother since she was a young girl. Teresa's mother would beat her, and Teresa would be the one who ended up apologizing. She shared the following example of a particularly intense gaslighting session: her mother had gotten upset with her because they were running late for church. Her mother began yelling at her in the car and cussing at her the whole way, accusing Teresa of being late on purpose because she didn't care about her mother and enjoyed upsetting her. Teresa had the audacity to tell her mother that it wasn't true and that she wasn't that type of person. This upset her mother even more.

"¿Cómo que no? ¿Quién te crees que eres, hija de tu chingada madre?" her mother yelled as she swerved the car into the 7-Eleven parking lot and told her to get out. Unsure of what to do, Teresa slowly unbuckled her seatbelt. Her mother swerved back into incoming traffic and yelled, "¿Qué chingados crees que estás haciendo? ¡¿Por qué te vas a bajar?!"

At this point, Teresa's body was shaking, and she began entering a state of learned helplessness. Her mind was beginning to disconnect from her reality and enter her mother's reality. It seemed like the only way to survive. Her mother gave her the silent treatment during the whole church service and the ride home.

During the silence, Teresa's mind was on overdrive: *What is she going to do when we get home? Did I really mess up so badly? Maybe I did make us late on purpose? Maybe I am as bad as she says. If I am as bad as she says, then I do deserve to be treated this way.*

On the car ride home, Teresa tried quieting her mind, but her mother's silent treatment made her thoughts grow louder and louder. As soon as they opened the door to their apartment, her mother lunged at her. Teresa fell to the ground after her mother's fist hit her right in the middle of her back.

"¡Mientras estábamos amarradas de la mano orando en la iglesia, yo estaba pensando en cómo te iba a partir tu madre!"

She looked her straight in the eyes as she said this. She lunged at Teresa and knocked her back to the floor with her fist. She lunged at her again, but this time her boyfriend held her back. Her mother was still yelling and trying to hit her again as Teresa army crawled into her room. She curled up in a corner crying until the following morning.

Teresa flinched reactively when her mother came into her room. "We both got a little out of hand yesterday. You made me feel like such a bad mother, and I had to show you that you can't talk to me like that. You can't treat me with such disrespect, especially on our way to church. Get dressed so we can go eat, and change that face of yours too. I better see you happy and smiling by the time we leave this house."

Teresa's head was spinning. "Sorry, mami," was all she could say.

Teresa learned to take the blame for others' wrongdoings. She learned that her feelings weren't worthy of being addressed and her boundaries were inexistent. Most of her life, she believed she existed to make others happy by saying and doing exactly what they wanted. If something goes wrong, it is her fault. She second guesses herself and her perception of reality. She fears speaking up for herself, because when she did, she was usually punished. Now, as an adult, she realizes she still feels like the scared little girl curled up in the corner, apologizing to the person who hit her.

I asked Teresa what she would tell that scared little girl who went to bed crying after crawling to her room that night. Her eyes got teary, and she whispered, "Que no fue su culpa."

Gaslighting tends to make us question and blame ourselves for things we didn't do and that someone else refused to take accountability for. It is a tool people use to disempower. We must use, find, and make the tools that empower, remind, and liberate us. One of the most powerful and most accessible tools we have is the power of our words. We can reclaim our thoughts, power, and essence with affirmations. I see affirmations as truths, invitations, reminders, and declarations. Oftentimes they are the things I need to hear but that no one is telling me, so I tell them to myself because they are too important to not be told (or said— even if I am the one to say them to myself).

NO FUE TU CULPA

Being told to not talk about what happened to you is a way of making you carry your story and suffering on your own. Self-silencing can turn into a sense of hopelessness that buries itself deep within our bones. We start believing nothing is going to get better because we don't deserve better. Learned helplessness is like a glue that keeps us stuck to the patterns of intergenerational trauma and abuse.

Learned helplessness occurs when someone experiences stressful events repeatedly without the ability to change or escape them. They learn that nothing they do helps them and therefore give up trying to change anything and simply accept their circumstances. Some people simply accept things are out of their control and normalize those feelings, or give up any hope for change. Others internalize it and assume it is what they deserve and that it is their destiny to live and die in such circumstances. Many children feel this learned helplessness and carry it with them into adulthood. They remain in abusive relationships because they learned early on these are things they cannot change or escape, so they feel they may as well accept them and think, Ni modo—así siempre han sido las cosas. Es lo que me merezco, y ya.

Psychologist Martin Seligman is credited with discovering this psychological phenomenon, which he first noted in dogs. Seligman and his team conducted an experiment in which dogs were put into constant shocking and stressful situations. Nothing they did changed their environment or the situations they were in. After some time, the dogs accepted their distressing circumstances, fell into depression, and gave up trying to do anything to change them. They observed similar patterns in humans.[9]

When we take into consideration the various forms of oppression and disadvantageous circumstances women are often born into, it is not shocking to hear many young girls and women adopt an attitude of learned helplessness early on. When you think about young girls born into abusive homes, poverty, dangerous neighborhoods, addiction, deportation threats, violence, etc., this state of learned helplessness is understandable and heartbreaking all at once. These are things outside of our control when we are little. There is little we could do to change them and little that could be done to change these circumstances. In most cases, there was little our parents could do to change certain things, such as their socioeconomic status, immigration status, etc. Our mothers most likely learned helplessness themselves from their mothers, and so on.

There is a beautiful thing called "learned hopefulness." It is when we (or someone close to us) teach ourselves how to hope. We begin to hope for better things when we believe we deserve better things. Part of this process requires us to want something better for ourselves and/or those we love. When we want something different than the circumstances we were born into, we begin to do things differently. Poco a poquito, we begin to imagine a different life, different circumstances, and even different ways of seeing ourselves. Learning to hope and believing we are worthy of beautiful things can be one of the most terrifyingly vulnerable and courageous things we do. Con heridas y todo. Con trauma y todo: mereces cosas bonitas, amor bonito, una vida bonita.

Yo estoy aquí para decirte: no fue tu culpa. You do not have to carry the weight of their shame. You are not responsible for what they did. You are not evil and there is nothing wrong with you. Your experience is valid. Necesitas sentir y llorar y gritar. Se vale enojarse. Your voice and your story and lived experience need to be shared, mujer. Maybe not with the world, but you cannot carry the silence within your tired bones all your life. Tienen que salir a respirar tus palabras, porque si no, te van a ahogar.

No fue mi culpa.

No fue mi culpa.

No fue mi pinche culpa.

Quiero decirte que tú no eras ni eres responsible por las heridas y acciones de tus padres. You are only responsible for yourself and who you are becoming despite where you come from. You were too small to know or do better back then. The only one responsible for themselves and for your well-being were your caregivers. Ahora, you are the one responsible for you. Y, ¿adivina qué? Tú puedes cambiar y puedes cambiar tus circunstancias.

You do not have to accept abusive, unsafe, or unloving circumstances. Porque mereces algo mejor, no chingaderas. Perhaps as a child you received the abuse inflicted by wounded adults who were irresponsible for their own wounds and actions. They were hurting, so they hurt you. You were a niña: vulnerable, confiada, y tal vez confundida as to what was happening or why they were treating you so badly. Now, you are a guerrera rising to her poder. You are realizing you have the agency, strength, words, and ganas de hacer las cosas de manera diferente, de sanar esas heridas, y de darte una vida diferente con un final feliz.

Part of your journey, mujer, includes you encountering who you were before trauma encountered you and choosing who you get to be after the trauma. I beg of you to not stay in the trauma, to navigate, swim, paddle, float, walk through it, but please do not build your house nor your identity there. You are so much more than your trauma. You are a badass who became and created beautiful things despite it.

Afirmaciones

I have everything I need to turn my life around. It is in my nature to give birth to new beginnings. My life is my masterpiece.
>*Tengo todo lo que necesito para cambiar mi vida. Es parte de mi naturaleza dar a luz nuevos comienzos. Mi vida es mi obra maestra.*

What's been done to me and what was taken from me does not define me.
>*Lo que me han hecho y lo que me han robado no me define.*

I am worthy of healing, peace, and love.
>*Yo merezco paz, sanación y amor.*

Nobody can take away my dreams, my will, my light, nor my strength.
>*Nadie me puede quitar mis sueños, mis ganas, mi luz ni mi lucha.*

I am using ancestral wisdom and strength to heal, build, restore. I am breaking the chains that oppressed them. I am continuing their legacy and picking up the torches they left behind.
>*Estoy usando sabiduría y fuerza ancestral para sanar, construir y restaurar. Estoy rompiendo las cadenas que los oprimieron. Estoy continuando su legado y prendiendo de nuevo el fuego que me dejaron.*

Chapter 6

Baking Bread

M any of us grow up on breadcrumbs because our mamis grew up on breadcrumbs because their mamis were also raised on breadcrumbs. We grew up malnourished and hungry. Whatever few breadcrumbs we got were called "love," and we believed it's what it was. However, as we grew up we got hungrier. These breadcrumbs weren't filling us up. We grew up seeing our mamis malnourished and chasing breadcrumbs in their relationships. Or they became so strong and hard that they convinced themselves they didn't need any breadcrumbs from anybody and were quietly starving themselves. We grew up surviving on these crumbs and either chasing them or learning to love starving ourselves.

How you form bonds with your friends, family, and romantic partners informs how you see the world, relationships, love, and yourself.

Your attachment style can provide information on your views on intimacy, the way you handle conflict, your views toward sex, your ability to communicate your wants and needs, and your expectations from your partner and relationships in general. This is pertinent to your identity development and how you relate to those around you because attaining the quality of the life you want relies on how you see yourself and how you interact with other people. Learning about your attachment style can help you understand more about who you are, how you are in relationship to others, and how you give and receive love. There are many different types of assessments that can help you determine your attachment style or the degree to which you identify with each attachment style, and we can display a little bit of each depending on the situation, environment, and person. The most important thing is that you are willing to look at and study yourself in an honest manner in order to know yourself on a deeper level.

The attachment we form with our caregivers also forms an important part of our identity and how we see ourselves and the people around us. We began to form our attachments desde que éramos bebés. This is because our developing brain can sense if our mother is in distress, if we are wanted, and if we are in danger. In the womb, our nervous system registers information about who we are and how we are coming into this world. Dr. Amir Levine and Rachel S. F. Heller, authors of *Attached: The New Science of Adult Attachment and How It Can Help You Find—And Keep—Love,* define attachment by the manner in which people receive and respond to intimacy in romantic relationships. According to Levine and Heller, there are four different attachment styles: secure, anxious, avoidant, and disorganized[1]:

- **Secure Attachment**: Secure attachment styles are characterized by healthy communication and emotional expression, the ability to express empathy in relationships, a balance of self-sufficiency and asking for help when needed, and the ability to set, maintain, and communicate boundaries. People with these attachment styles find it easy to establish new connections with other people without the fear or those people getting too close or leaving them.

- **Avoidant Attachment**: People with avoidant attachment style may be confident and independent, both in themselves and in their relationships with others, but avoid deeper emotional connections or vulnerability. Developing this attachment style may have been influenced by their childhood environment, in which expressing emotions was discouraged and hyper-independence was prioritized. People with this style may have difficulty fully trusting or opening up to other people, or themselves.

- **Anxious Attachment**: Anxiety is at the center of the anxious attachment style. Whether it's due to low self-esteem or past experiences, this attachment style results in behaviors like overthinking perceived threats, self-sacrificing to fit another person's standards, and the fear of abandonment.

- **Disorganized Attachment**: The disorganized attachment style can borrow the traits and characteristics of the avoidant and anxious attachment styles. There is a lack of cohesion when reacting in relationships due to emotional instability in childhood. That can result in people craving intimacy like in an anxious attachment, but moving away from it when received, like in the avoidant attachment style. People with this attachment style have learned to adapt and change their reactions to be better prepared for perceived emotional variables.

There are no right or wrong attachment styles. Our attachment styles simply reflect how we were cared for as a babies: if our parents were sensitive, available, and responsible, we'll most likely have a secure attachment style; if they were inconsistently responsible, we are likely to develop an anxious attachment style; and if they were distant, rigid, and unresponsive, we are likely to develop an avoidant attachment style. Our attachment styles in adulthood often reflect the attachment style we had with our caregiver, unless we have worked on building a new sense of self using different frameworks and styles of relating to our self and those around us.

Our attachment style plays an important role in how we choose our friends and partners. The people in our lives also inform our identity development, our self-perception, and our lived experience. If we pick partners who cannot or will not meet our needs or communicate effectively with us, we'll continue internalizing the belief that we are not worthy of healthy communication, amor del bonito, safe relationships, and partners who attune to our needs and value us as we deserve.

Ideally, we'd like to work toward building secure attachments with those we love and communicating our needs and wants effectively. We must know ourselves and have the ability to identify what we want and need in order to do so. When we develop a secure attachment to ourselves by being attuned to our needs and setting and respecting our own boundaries, establishing safe spaces and relationships for ourselves, and communicating our needs and emotions effectively, then it will be easier to develop secure relationships with others that affirm our sense of self, safety, and worthiness.

Building a secure attachment within yourself requires a willingness to unlearn old behaviors and establish new beliefs. This means learning to trust yourself and knowing that you can meet your own needs. The inner niña in you must have confidence that the adult you will take care of her, protect her, and not abandon her.

There are times during which we have to reparent ourselves in order to build a secure attachment with our inner child. We must mother ourselves and meet our essential needs: love, respect, safety, amor, confidence, and guidance. It is only when we do this that our inner child will bloom and heal the emotional wounds we've been carrying most of our lives. You will know you have created a secure attachment with yourself when you become a safe and trustworthy base for yourself, when you are attuned to your needs and can create the conditions necessary to feel confident and safe enough to pursue your interests and explore life. Secure people tend to be available, attuned to their needs, consistent, and encouraging. Securely attached people are usually more confident, know their worth, and know they deserve to be loved and valued at all times. Building a secure attachment is a sign of self-love and awareness, and you start to do this by having a sure sense of who you are as your own unique individual. It's why it is important for us to know who and how we are. Cómo estás y cómo eres y por qué eres como eres.

It is an act of faith in yourself and the people around you. It is a commitment to heal from past attachment wounds and learn new ways of seeing yourself, as well as giving and receiving love. You are setting yourself free by learning to trust yourself to grow, explore, and create.

As you learn about yourself, do so with the intention of loving every part of you. The healing process is not about perfection. It is not even about being the best version of yourself. It is about loving every part of you at every step of the process. La verdadera sanación no es la perfección. La verdadera sanación es aceptarte y amarte tal como eres mientras creces. Abrazarte cuando te caes y cuando te levantas.

Amarte con todo y a pesar de todo. Providing yourself with the love you need, especially in the moments when you feel most unlovable. This is building a secure attachment to yourself.

This largely depends on you becoming the adult your inner niña needed. Say it with me: "I am the adult my inner niña needed. I will give her everything she needs para florecer."

From this sense of security and peace with yourself, you will be able to build secure attachments with those around you. I love the book *How We Love, Expanded Edition: Discover Your Love Style, Enhance Your Marriage*, by Milan and Kay Yerkovich. In this book, the authors suggest that the way we love as adults is greatly influenced by how we were loved as children. This also gives way to how we love and are loved in relationships.[2] Essentially, you teach others how to love you, but first you need to learn how to love yourself. If you don't know how to love you or if you anxiously or avoidantly love yourself, it is most likely you will fall into relationships and attachments in which you feel insecure.

One of the most common insecure relationship patterns is the anxious-avoidant pattern in which one partner is anxious and the other is avoidant. These two types of people are usually drawn to each other because they each have what the other doesn't. The partner appears to offer what you inner niña was missing growing up. For example, when an avoidant person meets an anxious person, they are attracted by the attention, care, and kindness they receive. Avoidant people usually grew up emotionally starving and feeling neglected, dismissed, and ignored. Early on, they learned to care for themselves and be hyper-independent. The anxious partner's special attention and people pleasing tendencies offer them something they've been craving since they were little children. On the flip side, the anxious person is attracted to the avoidant person's sense of confidence, steady temperament, and strength. They feel validated for their people pleasing tendencies, since avoidant people are easy to fix, seemingly low maintenance, and tend to have low expectations. Most anxiously attached people grew up in chaotic, unstable homes, so this "stable and cool" avoidant person feels like a breath of fresh air. Initially, it feels like they both found what they'd always been missing.

However, when either of you is triggered, you most likely end up feeling as you did with your caregivers. The key is having a safe path back to repair. When one or both of you is insecurely attached, triggering or distressing times catalyze a pattern of chasing and distancing that sometimes deepens the attachment wound instead of repairing it.

The pattern usually goes as follows[3]:

1. The anxious partner is hypervigilant about pleasing their partner in order to receive the love and validation they crave.
   - They do everything they can to avoid upsetting their partner, avoid conflict, avoid rejection, and avoid feeling distance from their partner.
   - Their anxiety eases when they are making those around them happy.
   - They often minimize or dismiss their own needs, wants, and problems so they don't burden or bother anyone.

2. The avoidant person feels pressured by the anxious partner's need for reassurance and validation.

- They feel a bit invaded by the anxious person's need for closeness.
- They value independence and do not want the anxious person to encroach on their independence.
- They appear to lack empathy and crave distance.

3. The avoidant's need for space and independence triggers the anxious person, who interprets this as rejection, which makes them feel alone and in panic.
   - This propels the anxious person to try harder, hover more, and appease in order to get closer.

4. The anxious partner triggers the avoidant partner with their increased "neediness."
   - This causes the avoidant partner to create distance, detach, and evade emotions and time shared with the anxious partner.

5. The demand for distance poses a threat for the anxious person while serving as a protection for the avoidant.
   - The anxious partner tries to close the distance by capturing the avoidant person's attention and approval.
   - The anxious person becomes resentful, feeling they are giving more than they are getting.

6. The avoidant person becomes frustrated when the anxious person acts out.
   - They demand that the anxious person become more independent and may resort to disrespectful behavior, which pushes the anxious partner away.

7. This makes the anxious partner more hypervigilant and begins the cycle all over again.
   - Neither the anxious partner nor avoidant person gets their needs met, nor is their problem resolved.
   - There is no space or intention to repair the attachment wound. Rather, they are trying to protect themselves, while further deepening their wounds.

The only way to break this cycle is by learning how to bake a loaf of bread. When you learn how to bake yourself a loaf of bread, you will stop living off breadcrumbs. Anxiously attached people crave and chase the breadcrumbs, while the avoidant people starve themselves and refuse to share their breadcrumbs because they are afraid they will run out. Both end up hungry and malnourished. This all changes when we learn how to bake our own bread. When you learn how to bake a whole loaf of bread for yourself, you will stop chasing breadcrumbs. When you realize you can have an abundance of bread because you know how to make it for yourself, you won't worry about other people finishing off your breadcrumbs. You will trust and rely on your ability to bake your bread and feed yourself, and you can even share your bread with whomever you choose. This is what self-love and a secure attachment will provide for you: a life in which you can give yourself what you need while learning how to ask for and receive the love you want and deserve. You break the cycle when you develop a secure attachment with yourself. You develop a secure attachment when you are able to consistently and accurately identify, communicate, and meet your own needs.

Milan and Kay Yerkovich developed an illustration of what a secure attachment pattern could feel like. They call it the Comfort Circle[4]:

1. You begin by seeking awareness: self-awareness and awareness of your partner.
   • This requires time for self-reflection in order to understand feelings and underlying needs (yours and your partner's).
   • You engage in empathy and you notice when you and/or your partner are being triggered and need to be heard.

2. Engage with one another.
   • Healthy communication requires both partners to take turns being active listeners and speakers.

3. Explore each other's needs, story, and feelings.
   • Ask thoughtful questions that will bring clarity and help you gain a deeper understanding of your partner's emotions.
   • Validate the speaker's feelings even if you disagree.
   • Finish by asking the other: "What do you need?"

4. Resolution: effective communication, ask and receive.
   • The speaker makes a specific, reasonable request.
   • The listener meets their needs with actions and responses while being clear of what is within their capacity.

5. Aftereffects: completing the Comfort Circle will involve both people feeling heard and validated, and having their needs met.
   • This will increase trust, love, and bonding.

- The attachment wound will heal, and you will move more and more toward a secure attachment.
- This will encourage you to increasingly engage with the Comfort Circle rather than with the anxious-avoidant pattern.

Building that secure attachment is based not only on loving yourself—it requires you to trust yourself. Your inner niña is learning to trust the adult to meet her needs, care for her, listen to her, protect her, hold her, and love her. She needs you to apapacharla y nunca más abandonarla. You are learning to trust your voice, needs, boundaries, and capacity to love yourself. You are also learning to trust your future self and that the choices you make now will lead you to her and she will lead you to the most loving and healed version of you. Being a secure person also requires you to trust your ability to bake that bread.

Once you learn how to bake your own bread, you can share it with those around you without fear that it will run out. You know it is in your power to make more. You can share your bread with your mami and abuela and, better yet, teach them how to bake their own bread so they no longer have to survive off of breadcrumbs. It's time to stop surviving off of breadcrumbs, mujer.

Afirmaciones

I will embrace myself when I make mistakes, or else shame comes in. I am allowed to be imperfect. I am allowed to try again.

> *Cuando cometa errores me abrazaré, si no, entra la culpa. Tengo permiso de ser imperfecta. Tengo permiso para intentar las cosas de nuevo.*

I will not change myself for another. I worked too hard to find myself, build myself, and love myself back to life. I will protect the woman I've worked so hard to become and the one I am becoming.

> *No cambiaré por los demás. Trabajé demasiado para encontrarme, construirme y amarme hasta revivir.*
>
> *Protegeré a la mujer en la que he trabajado tanto por convertirme y en la que me estoy convirtiendo.*

There are days when I need to rise up. There are days when I need to rest. I will know which is which by listening to myself (mind, body, soul).

> *Hay días en los que necesito levantarme. Hay días en los que necesito descansar. Sabré cuál es cuál escuchándome (mente, cuerpo y alma).*

PART III

THE
BREAKTHROUGH

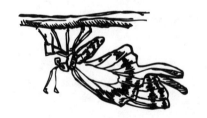

Chapter 7

Who the Fuck Are You?

Todo el mundo te quiere decir quién eres y cómo debes ser. The world will tell you who you are, si lo dejas. It's time to tell the world who you are, y no te dejes.

The majority of the time, women are not asked about who they are or what they'd like. We are told. They tell us who we should be and how we should be. There's a list of qualities dictating what "good" and "bad" women are. Ni nos preguntan; solo nos lo dicen.

"Women in the feminine mystique are not expected to grow up to find out who they are, to choose their human identity. Anatomy is a woman's destiny," say the theorists of femininity. "The identity of woman is determined by her biology."

It is assumed that by being born women, we are destined to follow one path. The path is pretty well paved and set out for us. Nos ponen en ese camino de toxic femininity desde que nacemos. They dress us in pink and tell us to like boys. Nos dicen que somos bonitas y frágiles. It feels like we are not allowed to decide who we are, that we have few options for who we can be. The ideas of femininity seem quite inflexible and established. We are often judged or condemned if we deviate from the oppressive cage of femininity and womanhood we are born into. I can almost write a list of rules I was told growing up, over and over again about how to be a "good woman," "una buena hija," y "una buena esposa," pero nadie me preguntó qué tipo de mujer yo quería ser. Nobody ever asked me what type of woman I wanted to be. I never asked myself. I simply did what I was told. I aimed to please the people around me as a survival mechanism. This is another rule for being a good woman: "Please the people." When we subscribe to this lifestyle of being a good woman, we are actually subscribing to toxic femininity.

When I say "toxic femininity" I'm referring to the concept of adhering to this rigid gender-binary societal standard of femininity and womanhood. It is a manifestation of internalized machismo. Toxic femininity upholds patriarchal systems and values. No seas una tóxica, mujer. You are oppressing yourself and the mujeres around you when you let them tell you what type of woman you should be. This is an invitation to stop trying to be a good woman. Porque en realidad te estás convirtiendo en una versión tóxica de feminidad que envenena el progreso de la liberación colectiva de las mujeres. Toxic femininity is a poison to the liberation of womankind—we want to move away from the binary, not uphold it. Be the type of woman you are. Be the type of woman who is free. Be whoever the fuck you want to be.

Yo quiero un mundo donde las mujeres puedan ser y hacer lo que les dé su chingada gana.

I want a world where women can be and do whatever the fuck they want.

See this as an opportunity to understand and love yourself a little more. Estúdiate. Ask yourself the questions you'd ask someone you were truly interested in getting to know. Take yourself on dates and reflect on your answers. Write them down. Take yourself in. Vas a encontrar algo hermoso.

I will provide some prompts for you to reflect on. Get a notebook just for these reflections, if you haven't already. Take your time answering them. There will be questions you may not know the answer to just yet. There are some that are obvious. Let yourself enter. Open up to yourself.

Society loves telling women who and how to be. It gives you a prescription for the paths you can take to be safe and accepted. Aguas a la que se atreva a desviarse. Ojo to those wild women who dare to pave their own path. You are taught to see yourself tied to your role to others. You are taught to see value in how you relate to and serve others. Whenever I would go to my mom's pueblo en Guadalajara, they'd refer to me as Kimberly, la hija de Mimi, la hija de Lula, la hija de Josefina, la esposa del Alacrán. They'd refer to their friends by their roles in their families and in society. Berta, la hija del carnicero. Maite, la de las tortas ahogadas. Lola, la trailera. The men just had their names or their nicknames: el Enano, el Chato, el Tomatón, el Gordo, etc. They just were, and that was enough. The goal is for you to be you and for that to be enough. Pero primero, you have to know who the fuck you are.

Quiero aclarar que it's not that associating ourselves with the things we do is bad. Calling ourselves a daughter, a wife, a mother, a partner, a student, a poet, an artist, or any other thing is not bad. Where the work comes in is in deciding what those labels mean to us and how we want to operate within them. Under the systems of racism, familismo, machismo, and marianismo, there are no choices—the rules are very well laid out as to which group has power over the other. But in reclaiming ourselves, you get to decide what kind of partner you want to be. You get to decide what kind of mother you want to be—if you'd like to become one at all. You get to decide what actions, decisions, and dynamics make up the role you choose to play. Perhaps you never asked yourself who you are, what you like, and why you are the way you are. Perhaps you never got to really know yourself because you were busy being who they said you should be in order to survive. Perhaps you don't know what you want because it never mattered in the spaces you were in. Perhaps you have felt out of control of your life your whole life. Maybe you haven't had the chance to learn what makes you happy, sad, mad, etc.

Many of us stop making decisions over our own lives as a trauma response. We feel powerless and helpless. So we simply throw up our hands and let others tell us what to do, how to do it, and who to be. Life in survival mode doesn't give us time to think about who we are. We are simply trying to get through the circumstances that we're in. We are simply trying to be. Desde que era niña I panicked whenever someone asked me about me. I hated those questions they always asked at school, church, or at the doctor's office: "What's your favorite…?" "Tell us three things about you." "How is your body feeling?" "What do you want?", etc. I hated and feared those questions because I didn't know the answers. As an adult, I still hated every time someone told me to tell them who I was or something about myself. I still didn't know the answers. I felt there was something wrong with me for not knowing anything about me. One time, when someone asked me what my favorite song was, I panicked because I couldn't even come up with one. So, I went home and studied my song list on my iPod and wrote down every single song I liked. I made a list of two hundred songs. Pa' la próxima ya sabré la respuesta. This is the reason behind the Get to Know Me exercise you are about to do. It is an opportunity for you to study yourself. It is imperative you have clarity and know exactly who you are. And once you find out who you truly are, you can love yourself.

One of the most important things you can do with your life is love yourself. You can have everything and everyone in the world, pero si no te amas a ti misma, te sientes vacía. You cannot truly and fully love yourself if you don't know who the fuck you are.

So, who the fuck are you, mujer?

Being able to answer this question and to love the answer you give is a sign of growth and self-liberation. Felicidades.

Here are some prompts to help get to know yourself a little better.

I invite you to take yourself out on a date and spend some quality time with you. Get to know yourself as if you were someone you were falling in love with.

I am . . .
- Write a list of all the things that make you you. Finish this sentence with as much information as you can.

I am not . . .
- Write a list of all the things you are not.

Favorite things
- Write lists of all your favorite things: music, food, movies, memories, people, etc.

Things I love about myself
- Write down as many things you love about yourself as possible.

Lista de miedos
- Write all the things you are afraid of. List all your fears (past, present, and future).

Lista de enojos
- Write all the things you are angry about or that can make you angry. How long have you carried this anger in your body and what does it feel like? How do you express it?

Lista de tristezas
- Write what makes you sad. What is the sadness you've carried in your life? For how long?

Lista de sueños
- Write down all the dreams you've ever had desde chiquita, from the dreams you think are silly and haven't shared with anyone, to your biggest dreams, which scare you.

You have to reclaim those parts of your essence that are perishing at the hands of machismo, homophobia, classism, racismo, and all the other bullshit oppressive systems in your life that have been dictating your identity. Tú puedes. Love those parts of you that society shamed you into believing were unlovable. I invite you to make yourself the main character of your own life.

Accepting what others tell us we should or shouldn't be is an act of self-betrayal and self-effacement. Self-effacement is the act of not claiming oneself, of letting oneself be eroded. When I think of this, I think of the coasts that become eroded by the sea. Shorelines do not move and slowly fade away as wave after wave hits them year after year. Many women live their lives slowly becoming eroded, smaller, dimmer versions of themselves as wave after wave of oppression hits them. I'd rather you be the ocean eroding the systems of oppression than the shoreline that gets eroded.

Enamórate de ti.

Enamórate de tus sueños.

Enamórate de tu libertad.

When we dream new dreams, we are planting the seeds for a different future. This future is distinct, and hopefully better than the past. Para que las cosas por fin cambien. Nosotras tenemos el poder de hacer las cosas diferentes a como siempre han sido. It starts with us, deep, deep within us. It starts with us choosing a name for ourselves and choosing loving things to call ourselves. We can identify ourselves however we choose to. Está en nuestro poder.

Think of a caterpillar who only sees itself as a worm and doesn't dare to believe it will one day be a butterfly. What if it still only sees itself as a worm even if when it finally gets its wings? It won't fly. Not because it doesn't have wings, but because it simply doesn't identify as a winged creature. It doesn't believe it is a butterfly. How you see yourself and your identity shapes how you take up space in this world.

See this as an opportunity to understand and love yourself a little more. Estúdiate. Ask yourself the questions you'd ask someone you were truly interested in getting to know. Take yourself on dates and reflect on your answers. Write them down. Take yourself in. Vas a encontrar algo hermoso.

Con cariño, siempre con cariño.

Afirmaciones

I am learning to rest and keep growing instead of giving up.
  Estoy aprendiendo a descansar para seguir creciendo en
  vez de rajarme.

I am a liberated, resilient, resistant badass—without shame.
  Yo soy una chingona libre, resistente y sin vergüenza.
  ¿Y qué?

I am learning to love all the things society taught me to hate
about myself.
  Estoy aprendiendo a amar todo lo que la sociedad me
  dijo que tengo que odiar de mí misma.

I embrace all the things that make me different, unique, and
beautiful.
  Yo acojo todas las cosas que me hacen diferente, única,
  hermosa.

I will take up space. I make the room more radiant with my
presence. I am no longer shrinking or hiding.
  Voy a ocupar espacio. Vuelvo más radiante el lugar con
  mi presencia. Ya no me voy a esconder ni a encogerme.

Chapter 8

Reclaiming Your Self

Kim Guerra is a name I gave to myself. It is not the name I was born with. I chose it. I was on the floor of our shitty Seattle apartment crying with my dog Chancho licking my tears. I don't know how long I was there. Probably hours. I had finally decided I would get a divorce. I couldn't afford a lawyer, so I had to DIY it. Grateful to have a printer at home, I held the thirteen warm sheets in my hand that I printed from the King County website. My birthday gift to myself would be getting them signed.

There was a section where I would forfeit my husband's last name and take on my old last name, or a new one. None of my old last names really fit me. One belonged to my siblings' dad, whom I'd lost connection with. My biological dad's last name didn't quite fit either. So I took my mom's maiden name: Guerra.

Kim Guerra.

It fit like a worn-in huarache. It felt like I had just fought a war for my life, my identity, and my freedom—and won. Guerra for the guerrera.

When the documents were finally signed, I took them to court and waited ninety days for the divorce to be finalized and my new name to become official. Impatiently, I waited for the judge to call my name on the day the court date finally came. "Kim Guerra." He reviewed everything, looked me up and down, and asked, "Are you sure?"

"Yes," I said.

"Well, then congratulations."

Sitting at the head of mi mami's dining table, I crossed my hands in front of me and announced, "I am officially divorced y ahora me llamo Kimberly Guerra. You can either support me or not, pero ya está hecho." This is how I began my birthday weekend. This was my breakthrough. It was glorious. There was such power to choosing my name, my path, my life. Es mía. Yo soy mía.

There is power in your name and how you choose to identify your-self. We have been called many names. Ada María Isasi-Díaz, author of *Mujerista Theology: A Theology for the Twenty-First Century*, tells us, "To name oneself is one of the most powerful acts a person can do. A name is not just a word by which one is identified. A name also provides the conceptual framework, the point of reference, the mental constructs that are used in thinking, understanding, and relating to a person, an idea, a movement."[1] Mujerista theology is dedicated to the liberation of mujeres. It is the opposite of machista. The mujerista theology takes into consideration the intersection of racism/ethnic prejudice, classism, and sexism. I was drowning in these societal systems and didn't realize it until I felt I couldn't breathe. I had given so many people, systems, and institutions power over my identity, I didn't know who I was anymore, nor who to be. Slowly, I started to reclaim myself and my power. Isasi-Díaz uses mujerista theology to "help us understand how much we have already bought into the prevailing systems in society—including religious systems—and have thus internalized our own oppression." Further, she states, "radical structural change cannot happen unless radical change takes place in each and every one of us."[2] Y sí, es cierto, mujer. Empieza dentro de nosotras.

I've met Latinas who are afraid to call themselves "feministas" because their countries have poisoned and ostracized the term and equated it to "man haters" and "feminazis." Being a feminist was seen as being a less desirable and and as a rebellious woman. In many cultures, it's treated as a dirty word. The independent woman was seen as a threat to the existing patriarchal systems in power. The self-identifying feminists were seen as man haters. I do not and will never identify as a man hater. I don't want to fuck them nor do I want to be them, but I see them with love as a fellow humans. They need to be part of the revolution. They need to heal their own wounds, caused by masculine oppression and machismo. This is the only way we will heal as a collective and transition into a less binary and more liberated society. "The feminists had destroyed the old image of a woman, but they could not erase the hostility, the prejudice, the discrimination that still remained. Nor could they paint the new image of what women might become when they grew up under conditions that no longer made them inferior to men, dependent, passive, incapable of thought or decision," shares Friedan in *The Feminine Mystique*.[3] Many of us grew up believing that being passive and incapable was our destiny. We grew up seeing the men, or even women themselves, treat women (and themselves) as if they were truly incapable of making decisions, accomplishing tasks, or thinking for themselves. When it came to important permissions or life decisions, I'd usually hear,

"Espérate a que llegue tu papá" or "Pregúntale a tu papá." We inherited a sense of uselessness and worthlessness. Any worthiness and value was intrinsically tied to the men in our lives. Sin ellos no éramos suficiente. A veces nos hacían sentir que sin hombres, las mujeres no eran nada; no podían sobrevivir even though we are the ones that gave birth, raised, fed, loved, and held these men from the moment they entered this world. Qué bonito que simplemente por nombrarse, las feministas pudieron crear una foto más bonita, más completa, de lo que significa ser mujer. This is one of the words I find refuge in because it is one of the only words which tells me that being a woman is enough, sufficient, y ya. Soy mujer y valgo por mí misma. No soy ni más ni menos que un hombre. I can stand on my own because I am my own human being, with my own identity and my own agency.

Lo más poderoso es saber que eres una mujer completa, reconocer tu poder y ver que no tienes límites—ni siquiera en cuanto a género. Si no quieres identificarte ni como mujer ni como hombre, ahora puedes. Si amas ser mujer, entra más en tu divinidad femenina. Si quieres ser hombre, entra en tu divinidad masculina. Si quieres ser los dos, o ninguno, o una combinación perfecta de los dos, dependiendo de lo que tu ser te pida, entra en tu esencia divina. Simplemente sé. Let yourself be your divine, complete, liberated self. Esto es una posibilidad que existe, y si no es una posibilidad para ti, vamos a luchar hasta que sea una posibilidad divina para todos nosotros.

Mujer. Poderosa. Queer. Chingona. Imparable.
Guerrera. Soft. Bad Bitch. My mother's daughter.
Bichota. Nalgona. Llorona. Berrinchuda. Empresaria.
Diosa. Tortillera. Maricona. Pinche. Lesbiana.
Lencha. Chismosa. Hocicona. Mujerona.

Take a moment to notice how you feel after saying these names out loud. Do you feel the power in your voice? Do you feel the strength emanating from your throat and into this universe as you speak life and truth into your life and existence? Do you feel the vibrations in your voice speaking a new reality into fruition? Are there new names you would add to this list?

How you see yourself and speak to yourself can change your life. Cada palabra es un color en tu obra de arte. Each word is a color in the masterpiece that is your life. You have the capacity to create something beautiful out of your life and your being. Do it, mujer. Do it, Badass Bonita. Esta es tu única vida. Este es tu único cuerpo. This is you. What are you going to make of yourself?

Decide. Hazlo. Vívelo. Transfórmate. Lucha. Créate. Renace. Date esas alas, mujer.

Decide. Do it. Live it. Transform yourself. Fight. Create. Be reborn. Give yourself those wings, woman.

It is time to name yourself, Badass Bonita. You can pick one name or a million. The important thing here is that you get to name yourself. You decided who you are and how you want to be in this world. If you choose to see yourself through an intersectional feminist lens and/or a mujerista lens, I encourage you to claim yourself as a mujer who is worthy of equality, security, liberation, and unapologetic joy. El objetivo no es lograr igualdad entre la mujer y el hombre. El objetivo es lograr igualdad y libertad sin género. Men are also being oppressed. No como mujer, ni como hombre, simplemente como humano. What type of human being do I want to be in this world?

I happen to be a human being who loves being a woman. You may be a human being who loves being nonbinary. Or a human being who is trans. What matters is being human. And you get to define that for yourself.

In my opinion, the most revolutionary and badass stage of metamorphosis is the breakthrough. Not many people dare to break out of the cocoon. It is where they feel safe and protected, and they never come out. They never get to experience their wings. It is in the cocoon that the caterpillar disintegrates in order to transform into a butterfly. Once it puts itself back together as a butterfly, it is ready to break through. The breakthrough is probably the most difficult and terrifying part. It means leaving the identity and world that you know and daring to step into who you were meant to become. It is breaking out of the old and stepping into the self you've transformed and chosen to be. ¡Atrévete a salir de tu capullo, mujer mariposa!

Ya es hora de que escribamos nuevas historias. Es hora de que nazca un nuevo tipo de mujer. Friedan states, "The New Women reflected the dreams, mirrored the yearning for identity and the sense of possibility that existed for women. And if the women could not have those dreams for themselves, they wanted their daughters to have them. They wanted their daughters to be more than the housewives, to go out in the world that had been denied to them."[4]

What dreams are we dreaming? What dreams have we inherited? What dreams are we fighting for and passing on?

Tus sueños valen la pena.

When we dream new dreams, we are planting seeds for a different future. This future is different and hopefully better than the past. Para que las cosas por fin cambien. Nosotras tenemos el poder de cambiar como han sido las cosas siempre. It starts with us, deep, deep within us. It starts with us choosing a name for ourselves and choosing loving things to call ourselves. We can identify ourselves however we choose to, está en nuestro poder.

Say this with me:

"I am a Badass Bonita."

"I am a human being giving myself wings through revolutionary self-love."

"I will have the courage to break through and fly."

Afirmaciones

I look in the mirror and see a warrior woman. I see a woman who has fought for her life and won. I see a woman determined to keep fighting for herself, for all mujeres, and for her people. I see a mujer I am proud of. I see a butterfly learning to use her wings. I see someone I love.

> *Cuando me miro en el espejo veo a una mujer guerrera. Veo a una mujer que ha luchado por su vida y ha ganado. Veo a una mujer decidida a luchar por sí misma, por otras mujeres y por su gente. Veo a una mujer de la cual estoy orgullosa. Veo a una mariposa aprendiendo a usar sus alas. Veo a alguien a quien amo.*

I choose how others treat me by how I treat myself. I choose to be powerful and strong in my self-love. I choose to be soft, intelligent, and courageous. I can be whoever and however I want. I have the power to choose.

> *Yo escojo cómo voy a dejar que me traten los demás. Yo elijo ser poderosa y fuerte en mi amor propio. Yo elijo ser tierna, inteligente y valiente. Yo puedo ser quien y como yo quiera. Yo tengo el poder de escoger.*

I am like the butterflies—I give myself wings.
> *Soy como las mariposas: me doy alas a mí misma.*

I am my own genre of mujer. I make my own rules. I will no longer fit into boxes created to oppress me.
> *Yo soy mi propio tipo de mujer. Yo hago mis propias reglas. Ya no me meteré en las cajas creadas para oprimirme.*

Chapter 9

See Yourself with Eyes of Love

What does it mean to be a liberated mujer who loves herself? What does it mean to be a Badass Bonita?

It means that you are committed to the woman you are becoming. It means you are committed to your metamorphosis and to your wings. Que no te vas a quedar calladita, ni haciendo las mismas cosas de siempre. Tú vas a volar. You will love yourself enough to become a mujer con alas. Self-love is not perfection. It is more than acceptance. It is an intentional commitment to yourself: your healing, your growth, your wings, your expansion, your light, your voice, your truth, your story, your essence, and your becoming. Your roots, your cultura, tu idioma, tus tías criticonas, tu rancho, tu barrio, tu comida, tus canciones—all of those things are components of who you are, mujer. Son cosas pequeñas, pero merecen amor. I want you to love yourself so well that you know los detallitos de ti y que te tomes el tiempo para darles amor.

When I think of self-love, I think of ugly crying and mocos running down my face. I feel the llanto in my chest que viene de las profundidades de mi alma. Self-love isn't pretty. It isn't Instagrammable, nor can you put a filter on it. It is in the moments in the desert where you find yourself tirada en el piso, abandonada, sucia, desesperada, full of shame, greñuda, con una tristeza que no te cabe en los ojos. It is in this moment when you scoop yourself up in your arms and you love that version of you—the one you don't want anyone else to see. The one shame tells you is unlovable. You cry with her. Le haces caricias en su carita wet with tears que no dejan de caer como ríos de dolor y sufrimiento. You hold her shaking body and assure her you are not going anywhere. You listen to her as she shares her shame, secrets, trauma, pain. You listen. You do not judge. You see her with unconditional love. You tell her you love her a pesar de todo lo que ha vivido, hecho, lo que le han hecho a ella. You love her in her wildness. You love her toda mocosa y sucia. You promise to take care of her and heal her wounds. Sus heridas, su sangre, su corazón destrozado. You do everything in your power to make sure she stops bleeding. You bathe her and bring her to a safe place. You show her how beautiful and powerful she is. You hold her when she is scared to speak up and try new things. You fight for her and go in the shadows with her. You remind her of her light. You do not shame her or control her or try to put her in any boxes. You let her be who she is right in that moment, and you simply love her. You let her tell you everything about herself.

Getting to know her is also an act of love. Así. When there is love and acceptance like this, there is a deep knowing and understanding that we are in the process of becoming. In those moments, even though you may not see them, you know it is part of the process for getting your wings. They are on their way. You are a work of art in process. Una mariposa en su metamorfosis. You are not going to stay tirada en el piso forever. Pero you have to love yourself there and you also have to love yourself enough to choose to rise from there. You have to love yourself enough to commit to the process of your healing. You are becoming.

Self-love and self-care both matter, but they are not the same. We often think they are interchangeable, pero no es así. Self-love is the act of planting the seeds and self-care is the act of ensuring these seeds grow. Self-love goes deep. Self-love is the commitment and faith in your growth and worthiness. Self-love is not about perfection. It's not even about being the highest self or the healthiest version of you. It's about choosing to love yourself even at your worst, especially at your worst. It's not about your performance or appearance. It is about who you are. Your essence. Your soul. It is about being enough in every way, any day, every part of who you are. It is a knowing and a deep-rooted commitment to loving oneself unconditionally. Self-love is loving yourself enough to change and heal even if it is uncomfortable and has you ugly crying in your room. Self-love is holding yourself accountable and being responsible for your actions. Self-love requires discipline. Self-love requires all of you. It isn't a surface level exercise or something you check off a to-do list. It is a lifelong journey. It is a lifestyle. It informs every decision you make. Sometimes self-love looks like asking ourselves this question about everything: Is this loving to me?

Self-love often looks like asking ourselves what the most loving thing we could do for ourselves is and doing it over and over again. A pesar de todo. Self-love means doing whatever it takes to give yourself the life you deserve, to stop the bleeding, to heal the wounds, to break the cycles, to go after your dreams, to give yourself a chance to do things differently, to believe in yourself, to treat yourself kindly and with compassion, to go to therapy, to eat your vegetables and drink your water, to take yourself dancing, to surround yourself with good people, to be present, to breathe deep, to cry, to stand up for yourself, to hold yourself, to set boundaries, darte abrazos apretados, to forgive yourself, to rest, and simply to be and believe you are being—all because you love yourself. Nada más y nada menos.

Self-care is also important. It is a manifestation of the love that you have for yourself. You care for yourself because you love yourself. Te cuidas porque te amas. Te amas y obviamente te cuidas. Self-care can look like doing practical things like taking yourself to the doctor, exercising, journaling, meditating, and putting on one of those face masks in the bathtub. It can look like buying yourself flowers, treating yourself to a fancy dinner, or simply respecting your night and morning routine. Self-care also has to do with believing you are worthy of respect and care. You were not created to spend your whole life taking care of others and not taking care of yourself. Es hora de soltar esa idea. You were created for so much more. You deserve care and rest and joy. Cuídate como si fueras tu flor favorita, mujer. Care for yourself as if you were the most valuable person in your life—because you are. You are not selfish for taking care of yourself. You are not doing anything wrong for taking time for yourself and making yourself a priority.

Self-care can sometimes feel intimidating, especially if no one taught you how to do it. Or if you were shamed for wanting to take care of yourself. I've made a list of ways you can take care of yourself. You can add to it as you gain practice, for self-care is also a practice. It is something you do for yourself that comes more naturally as time goes on. Consider some of the practices below when curating your self-care ritual:

The Bad Bitches with Soft Hearts Take Care of Themselves List

- Create a morning routine. (Set a wake-up time and activities that are a nourishing way to start your day.)
- Wake up and don't pick up your phone.
- Meditate.
- Journal.
- Write down what you are grateful for.
- Say your affirmations out loud while looking in the mirror.
- Prepare a healthy, nourishing meal for yourself.
- Take a bubble bath.
- Take five deep breaths.
- Create a loving way to connect with your body through movement (yoga, dance, working out).
- Buy yourself flowers.
- Take a walk.
- Take yourself on a date.
- Create a vision board.
- Declutter your space.
- Read a self-help book.
- Schedule time with friends.
- Cook your favorite meal.
- Do things and spend time with people that inspire you.
- Take a social media break.
- Spend time in the sun.
- Drink water.
- Watch the sunrise and/or sunset.
- Take time to do nothing.
- Call/text someone you love.
- Try something new.
- Get your nails done.
- Get a massage.
- Create art.
- Learn a new skill (crochet, embroidery, hula hooping).
- Do something your inner niña would like.
- Eat your favorite snack.
- Sit in the sun.
- Volunteer your time.
- Listen to a podcast.
- Give yourself a facial.
- Plan a getaway.
- Join a support group.
- Get aromatherapy.
- Prende una velita.
- Unfollow people who don't add to your life.
- Sit in silence.
- Ponte a limpiar y pon tu playlist de señora favorita.
- Stay in.
- Go out.
- Do whatever you want without asking anyone for permission.
- Haz lo que te dé la chingada gana.

All of these are essential elements to your becoming, mujer mariposa. Use them. Take them like the medicine they are. Let them show you your becoming. Hold on to them for dear life. Transform them. Let them transform you. Conviértete en el amor de tu vida.

Loving and caring for yourself requires commitment. Be willing to do and give everything it takes for you to get your wings. Many of us have already given our vows to another person. We have committed to love and to be there for the other. However, we mustn't forget that our relationship with ourselves is the most important one. How are you going to love, care, and empower yourself from this day forward as long as you shall live?

When I got married, I wrote my own vows. It was a sacred process that I did not take lightly. I meant every word when I wrote it. I was willing to commit my whole life to another person. I was willing to go through everything by his side. However, at that point in my twenty-two years of life I had no idea who the fuck I was. I did my best to uphold those vows. I gave everything until there was nothing of me left to give. When I left that marriage, I realized I had no idea who I was. How could I commit so fully to someone else when I was so disconnected from myself? How could I love another when I had no idea how to love me?

We are so ready to give ourselves away to others, but we are still learning to give ourselves the same love and commitment. We will be doing that today.

It's time to write vows to yourself.

These vows are a promise to yourself, your inner niña, the woman you are today, and the woman you are becoming. Take time to vow to yourself how you will dedicate your life to loving you. This is self-love. Take time to write how you will love, protect, nurture, care for, fight for, and honor yourself (mind, body, spirit, soul). Vow to choose yourself and promise yourself to hold you with compassion through sickness, health, richer, poorer, tears, laughter, and all of life's adventures. Vow to do everything in your power to make sure you heal, grow, and become the woman of your dreams. Vow to be the most beautiful version of yourself and give yourself the love you deserve. If you have a higher power, include them in your vows and ask for a blessing of this sacred relationship between you and your soul, your inner niña, and the woman you're becoming.

Promise to trust and be faithful to yourself, your dreams, your needs, your values.

Once you are done writing your vows, you will do a visualization and read them out loud to yourself in the mirror.

I want you to visualize what we are about to do as if it were a sacred ceremony between you and your future self. You will be making a commitment to her: to love her, hold her in sickness and in health, for richer and for poorer, through it all. You will be by her side, loving her, caring for her, giving her all she needs to get the love and life she deserves.

Find a comfortable spot and close your eyes. You can place your hands in your lap, across your stomach, or over your heart. Feel the way your chest rises and falls with each breath and notice how your body unwinds. If there are any thoughts that cross your mind—things you have to still do or random pieces of information—let them pass. Visualize your future self standing across the altar from you. This visualization will guide you through a sacred commitment you are making to your highest self. This is to be taken with the reverence we give to holy matrimony. Oftentimes we commit our lives and make vows to others, yet we abandon ourselves. I believe that the relationship we have with ourselves should be the most intimate, loving, and enduring one. So, as you get ready to write these vows, light a candle, buy yourself flowers, burn some palo santo, and truly take this time to connect con tu alma preciosa. Read them to yourself in the mirror. What are the two of you wearing? Who is sharing the space with you? What do your surroundings look like? Are there flowers? Decorations?

If you want the ceremony to just be between the two of you—you get to decide. You can also have your inner niña there as the flower girl or standing next to the woman you're becoming at the other end of the altar. This is your time. The ceremony of your dreams, binding you to the person that will be with you always—you. Celebrate. In your visualization, have as much cake as you want. Dance with yourself until your feet hurt. Give yourself the gifts you've always wanted. Cherish the moment you make this agreement with yourself.

Vows to the Woman You Are Becoming

Think about the life you want and visualize the woman you are becoming:
- What does she look like?
- Where does she live?
- What is her energy like when she walks into a room?
- How does she feel about herself?
- What does her morning routine look like?
- What does she dress like?
- What type of relationships does she have?
- Who are her friends?
- Where does she work?
- How does she spend her time?
- What are her hobbies?
- Where does she go for fun?
- Where is she traveling to?
- What goals is she working toward?

- What is she most proud of?
- How is her heart feeling?
- What negative cycles has she broken?

Once you have a clear picture of what your future self looks and feels like, I want you to visualize yourself walking toward her down the aisle. Look at her with eyes of love and let her look at you with eyes of love and gratitude for every choice you made that contributed to her becoming. When you feel ready, take a deep breath and read them out loud to her–to you. Mark this day on your calendar. It is sacred. It is your commitment day: to your wings, to your becoming, to being a Badass Bonita, to yourself.

Below, you'll find an example love letter to the future woman I'm transforming into. I encourage you to write one of your own.

A love letter to the woman I'm becoming:

I make my decisions thinking of you.
I am healing so you can know what it's like to be free. Eres mi prioridad.
I want to remind you: tienes alas.
Cada día brillas más.
You are becoming a more beautiful version of yourself. Te admiro for not giving up. I'm excited to see you glow y vivir la vida que siempre soñamos. Te amo, mujer mariposa.
Mujer guerrera.
Eres tierna. Protect your softness.
Tu manera de ser es mágica.
Eres fuerte y estás aprendiendo a ser más vulnerable. When you feel like you are too much, remember you've fought

hard to become every bit of who you are. You are a bad bitch. Please, don't shrink for anyone.

You are meant to shine bright.

Tu luz y tu corazón are one of the most powerful things about you. I vow to help you see your own beauty and power every day.

I vow to love you con ganas y sin miedo.

Even when it gets hard, through it all, voy a estar contigo. Prometo verte con ojos de amor y tratarte y hablarte con cariño. Darte el amor que te mereces: amor del bueno, amor bonito.

Eres tierna. I vow to protect your softness.

Tu manera de ser es mágica. Prometo tomar decisiones y rodearte de gente que te ayude a brillar más.

I vow to believe and remind you of your worthiness so you can pursue, accomplish, and dream bigger dreams. No nos vamos a encoger ni detener por nada ni nadie.

I vow to help you see your own beauty and power everyday.

I vow to hold you.

I vow to dance and laugh as much as I can in this life.

I vow to enjoy your company and do things with only you in mind.

Sobre todo, prometo no abandonarte jamás.

Esta vida la dedico a amarte en alma, mente, cuerpo, corazón y espíritu.

All of these are essential elements to your becoming, mujer mariposa. Use them. Take them like the medicine they are. Hold on to them for dear life. Transform them. Let them transform you. Conviértete en el amor de tu vida.

Thank you for committing to loving yourself. Thank you for committing to the process of becoming. You are creating a masterpiece with this life you've been given. Your voice is changing lives: starting with yours. You get to decide who and how you become the mariposa you were destined to become—mujer con alas, Badass Bonita, guerrera. How you become is important. The tools you use to become are essential. The art of becoming isn't a magic trick that happens with the wave of a wand. The art of becoming is an act of love and metamorphosis. Es tu propia revolución.

Te mereces cosas bonitas. Aprende a recibirlas.

When you look back at this time, you're going to be so grateful you chose you.

Your future self will thank you for committing to your healing and for learning to love yourself.

Revolutionary love will be your legacy.

Listen to your divine calling.

Take a moment to thank yourself for showing up for yourself and for having the courage to commit to yourself. Not many people make it past the breakthrough stage. Not many people have the courage to give themselves wings and actually use them.

Tienes alas, mujer.

You are ready to fly.

Es la hora de volar:

con ganas y sin miedo.

Your life and heart are far too divine for you not to make them into something beautiful.

Your wings are yours.

No one can take them away from you.

Make this life your masterpiece.

Tú eres tuya.

Ámate con ganas.

Afirmaciones

The most powerful beings in the world are women who love themselves. I am one of those women.

> *Los seres más poderosos del mundo son las mujeres que se aman. Yo soy una de esas mujeres.*

I will stop making excuses to not respect myself. I am capable. I will create beautiful things. I will drink water. I will laugh loudly. I am growing and glowing. I will value the beauty my soul has to offer this universe.

> *Dejaré de poner excusas para no respetarme. Soy capaz. Crearé cosas hermosas. Tomaré agua. Me reiré fuerte. Estoy creciendo y brillando. Valoraré la belleza que mi alma le ofrece a este universo.*

I look at myself with eyes of love. I see my strength. I see my beauty. I see my resilience. I see the battles my ancestors fought. I see my healing. I finally see me.

> *Me miro a mí misma con ojos de amor. Veo mi fuerza. Veo mi belleza. Veo mi resistencia.*

Mujer, I will protect you, look out for you, and fight for you.

> *Mujer, te protegeré, me encargaré de ti y lucharé por ti.*

PART IV

USING YOUR WINGS

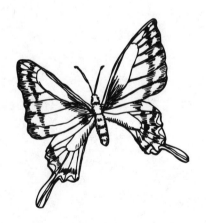

Chapter 10

Fight the Shame
and Set Boundaries

"Sinvergüenza" is a term we use to insult someone—especially women. It means "without shame" and implies women should have shame and that women without shame should be ashamed of themselves. Shame is suffocating. Shame is what they use to silence us. Shame is a poison they force us to drink desde que somos niñas. By the time we are adults, we are covered in shame, overflowing. We almost believe it is who we are supposed to be. Shame does not have to be a part of your identity. It is what is keeping you from being free.

There is a dance between vergüenza y vulnerabilidad. May vulnerability always lead. When vulnerability leads, vergüenza follows and realizes maybe it shouldn't be taking up too much space. In this chapter, we will begin by dancing with shame. We will get to know her and see how much space she has taken up in our identity and life. We will observe the dance between shame and vulnerability. Then, we will ask vulnerability to dance and we will follow. We will explore the connection between shame, vulnerability, and silence.

Finally, there's the Fuck Being Calladita lifestyle. It is an invitation to unsubscribe from shame and self-silencing and subscribe to a life in which you are free to love, say, do, think, and be whoever the fuck you want—anything but calladita.

One of the leading voices on shame and vulnerability is Brené Brown. Her work has revolutionized how we see vulnerability as a strength rather than a weakness. Shame is an option rather than a lifestyle or destiny. Shame is what stops us from being vulnerable. According to Brown, "Vulnerability is the birthplace of love, belonging, joy, courage, empathy, and creativity. It is the source of hope, empathy, accountability, and authenticity." Vulnerability is the balm that dissolves the sting of shame. It allows us to show ourselves in an authentic way and trust those we are sharing with to love us and receive us with compassion. By sharing our voices, thoughts, and stories, we create connections that fight the isolation of shame and silence. Shame lives off of silence. So does abuse. When we choose to break that silence, we are directly choosing to fight the shame which told us our voice was not important or that our story shouldn't be heard. Shame has such a dangerous effect on our lives. It often feels like a hand gripping our neck. Sometimes it gets so heavy people try finding different ways to cope with it. Brown's research tells us shame is highly correlated with addiction, violence, disease, aggression, depression, eating disorders, and bullying. It is a poison which destroys us and those around us.

I witnessed shame consume the women in my family. They were envenenadas por su pena y odio hacia sí mismas. I'd hear how they talked about their bodies and other women's bodies. I'd hear them fat shaming and slut shaming and spreading shame everywhere because they were overflowing with it. The shame was oozing out of them and they didn't know how to stop it. Shame controlled them and infused their every word. It was on the seasoning of our food. It was in our hair. It was everywhere. I couldn't escape it. It was controlling us all while we were trying to control everything and everyone. They would criticize themselves and every other woman they saw. Hasta los dedos de los pies les criticaban. They too would find reasons and places to inject shame. We were busy finding everything that made us unlovable based on what society and trauma had instilled in us. Then, we would go and find what made other people unlovable to make ourselves feel a little better. However, it would only make us feel worse. Shame can be an endless cycle of poison breeding poison. We need the medicine. We need to uproot the seeds of shame and unsubscribe from the shame-filled lifestyle. I want to spread medicine over my wounds, not shame. I want to offer medicine, not poison, to the women who surround me. We have all suffered enough.

Shame makes us forget how fucking incredible we are. It sucks our light and makes us feel like a monster living in the shadows. It is a dark force with the sole purpose of keeping us from loving ourselves, receiving love from others, and giving love. Shame tells you all the shitty things about you. It blinds you to your own beauty. Its voice can get so loud it deafens you to your own voice and to the voice of love. When I think of the people I love, I am not actively looking for their imperfections or for reasons to hate them. I am not looking for their mistakes or seeing the places they failed. Their imperfections make me love them more because it is part of what makes them unique. It is part of who they are. I don't get to pick and choose the parts of them to love. I love all of them. I accept them as they are, not for how I think they should be. When they make mistakes, I forgive them for we are human and we all fuck up. It doesn't make them a fucked up human who is unworthy of my love. They are a human I love who fucked up and that fuckup will not change my love for them. There are moments I see people I love and my heart wells up with all the love I have for them. Seeing their smile or hearing them laugh makes me happy. Their joy is my joy. Their existence brings me joy. I thank God they exist and for their presence in my life. I thank God for the light and beauty they bring to this world and my life. I celebrate who they are. I love them when they are being raw and vulnerable—when they are not performing or pretending. This is the beauty of love and human connection. It is what keeps us alive. Shame keeps us from being able to give this to ourselves or to receive it from others. Imagine looking at yourself in this way. Imagine seeing yourself with eyes of love instead of with eyes of shame. Imagine seeing the beauty and light your existence brings to this world. Life without shame allows us to do that. With shame it is impossible.

Vulnerability is medicine. It can also feel absolutely intimidating. My therapist is an older Colombian woman. She reminds me of the grandma from chocolate Abuelita. Her voice is gentle and kind. Her hair is gray. She is a little fluffy. Her eyes are soft, profound. She knows how to hold me, and most importantly, how to help me hold myself. Dr. María is also excellent at seeing through my bullshit. During a particularly difficult session in Oaxaca, she stopped me and looked at me. Then she said, "You've been hiding your whole life. Even though parts of your life are very public, you only show people what you want them to see. You don't want them to see all of you. You are afraid to show the real you: the Kim that's not always smiling. Es tiempo de quitarte tu armadura. No siempre tienes que ser una guerrera. A veces simplemente debes ser humana." We then did inner child work and visualization in which I had to choose to stop hiding and pretending to be strong. She asked me if I remembered when I first put on my armor. The memory came to me instantly.

My first "real" job was a summer program my middle school offered where we would "beautify" the city. It was called something like "Clean & Green" and it was created to keep kids out of trouble. Our parents would drop us off at the Taco Bell parking lot and a white van would come and pick us up. We would go around the city and pick up trash, plant trees, and paint over graffiti. It was fun and gave us something to do in the long summer months. There was a boy I had a crush on named Santiago. His grandpa and my mom were usually the last ones to pick us up. We would wait for them under the shade of a tree in the Taco Bell parking lot. I'd tease him because he was so shy. "Soy serio como mi abuelo," he'd say. He talked to me about how his parents were gone, and his grandparents took care of him. I didn't really share much about my family. One day, he looked at me and stayed quiet for a long time. Then he said, "Tienes ojos tristes. Cuando piensas que nadie te ve, dejas de sonreír y te ves triste como esas niñas que están tristes porque alguien las violó." Goddamn it, Santiago! I felt exposed. He was right. I did hide my sadness behind my smile. From that day forward, I was always smiling. It was my armor. I didn't want anyone to see my sadness or think of me as one of those girls con un caso triste de *La Rosa de Guadalupe* (a novela which showcased "real life" cases of tragedy and how things changed magically with the miracles from la Virgen de Guadalupe). So I smiled and hid. By the time I got to high school, I was an expert at hiding myself. I'd dress up and look good, so that people would think I was good. They didn't even have to ask how I was doing—just look at me! I was wearing heels everyday. My hair was always done. My outfits always matched. I was on time. Straight As and AP courses. Honors program and extracurriculars were added to my arsenal. I'd spend some time with friends but always kept them at a distance. They couldn't get too close. They knew just enough about me, but never enough to actually get to know me. They knew the version of me I wanted them to know. The rest of the time I'd go to the library to study, write, or read my Bible. By that time, I began to get heavily involved in church. This did not help my shame-filled lifestyle. It added to my shame and my guilt and my drive for perfection. I wanted to please God, the pastor, be a good daughter, and become the modern Proverbs 31 woman they were always preaching about at church. I needed to be perfect. It was the only way they would love me. They couldn't know I was a sad girl who was molested by her stepdad, who didn't eat because she hated her body and was terrified of losing control, who weighed herself obsessively, who didn't have close friends because she was afraid of the closeness, and who smiled to hide the sadness in her eyes. I perfected the art of hiding and silencing myself. It got to the point that I believed it myself. My armor became my second skin. I didn't know how to live without it. I was terrified of taking it off. More so, I was terrified of what I'd find behind it. So, I didn't until that day in therapy with Dr. María.

She saw right through it and she gently helped me take it off. We went through the layers and layers of armor and masks I'd put on. The shame I was carrying was profound. I made the choice to take it off and let myself be human. I chose vulnerability. I chose to feel all my feelings. I embraced my imperfections and gave myself permission to make mistakes. I took the weight of perfection off my shoulders. Perfection does not exist. It is a set up for failure and a cruel illusion created by shame. Perfection is a lie. It is not a human condition. By definition it is inhumane. By taking off the armor of shame, I chose love. I felt naked. I was terrified. It felt like showing up naked to the first day of school. After the therapy session ended, I went to the hotel room and covered myself up in the blankets. I felt like a scared little girl. I was shaking, crying, and terrified. I didn't want to leave. I felt like I couldn't. Encuerada. Sin (la armadura de la) vergüenza. How the fuck do people live like this? I knew I couldn't have survived without my armor back then, but now I was in a safe enough place to try. So, I did. I went outside in the colorful streets of Oaxaca without my armor for the first time. Believe it or not, I felt like I was seeing the world and myself with different eyes. Ojos sin vergüenza.

I stopped trying to hide the sadness in my eyes. I let it out gently, one tear at a time. I finally let myself cry. Trying to be strong and fearless had actually made me numb for many years. My feelings were inaccessible after I put on my armor. Without it, it felt like my heart started to thaw. I began to feel. There were times I didn't have the tools to deal with my feelings and I'd feel overwhelmed. It all felt so raw. Pero poco a poco mi corazón y mi mente se fueron acostumbrando. Una lágrima a la vez.

Vulnerability extends its hand and lovingly teaches us to dance. Sometimes people think being vulnerable is like jumping out of a plane. It doesn't have to be like that. It can be gentle and slow. It gives you the space and safety for softness. When we lead with vulnerability, or better yet, let vulnerability lead us, we enter into a place of connection and authenticity. This is a place of strength and intentional surrender. Just like love cannot coexist with abuse. Love cannot exist without vulnerability. In *All About Love*, bell hooks shares, "We cannot know love if we remain unable to surrender our attachment to power, if any feeling of vulnerability strikes terror in our hearts."

Abuse is all about power, and control. It thrives in shame infused silence. Love is all about vulnerability, acceptance, and care. It may be time to reexamine your definition of love. bell hooks reminds us, "An overwhelming majority of us come from dysfunctional families in which we were taught that we were not okay, where we were shamed, verbally and/or physically abused, and emotionally neglected even as we were also taught to believe that we were loved. For most folks it is just too threatening to embrace a definition of love that would no longer enable us to see love as present in our families. Too many of us need to cling to a notion of love that either makes abuse acceptable or at least makes it seem that whatever happened was not that bad." Many of us grew up receiving abuse in the name of love. Now, as adults, we struggle because there is an internal dissonance when it comes to love. How is it that the people who claim to love me the most are the ones who hurt me the most? They may have called it tough love. Maybe because it wasn't love. Maybe it was just tough. Love lead by vulnerability leads us to softness. When someone meets our vulnerability with empathy and kindness, the shame dissolves. Our heart finds a safe place to land, expand, and be soft. I think love is found in the people and places where our hearts can take off their armor. We cannot get to those places and people without the vulnerability acting as the light guiding us forward. Trust in the softness. Trust in your capacity to love and be loved. Our society has taught us to fear vulnerability and see it as a weakness. It is the medicine that cures the shame. It is stronger than the shame which oppresses us all. Softness is not weakness. It is easy to be hard and tough in this world. Only the brave dare to be soft. I have fought hard and peeled back many layers to get my softness back. Vulnerability was terrifying at first, but it set me free. La vulnerabilidad me invitó a bailar and taught my heart soft love. It let my soul breathe once again after being suffocated under the armor of shame, which I believed was keeping me safe.

What kept me safe were the boundaries I learned to set once I took off my armor.

Boundaries are a form of self-love. It is how you teach others how to love you by how well you love yourself. It is a form of establishing safety for yourself and those around you. It is hard to become the most badass, beautiful version of yourself without boundaries. I will go as far as saying you cannot love yourself if you cannot establish healthy boundaries. This can be really intimidating, especially for those of us who grew up in a culture in which there is not really a word for boundaries nor are they normally encouraged. I remember the first time I tried to set a boundary my mom responded with, "¿Y tú quién chingados crees que eres? ¡A mí no me vas a decir cómo tratarte o cómo hablarte o nada de eso, si yo te parí!" I considered never setting a boundary again after that response to my first try. Therapy helped me understand why they were important and how significantly my life (and I) would change once I began setting boundaries that created safe and loving relationships and environments for myself.

Usually, creating healthy boundaries leads to feeling safe, loved, calm, and respected. They are an indication of how you allow people to show up for you and how you show up for others. Ultimately, it is a reflection of how you show up for yourself.

The lack of boundaries often leads to chaos and you doing everything for everyone except yourself. It is hard to evolve and progress in your self-love journey when you are busy taking care of everyone else's needs. Our cultura usually praises women who do this. We are raised to take care of everyone and everything else. If you take time for yourself, say no, o si no le prestas dinero a la vecina de la madrina de tu tía they will call you selfish and maleducada. When this happens, practice the mantra, "Me vale madre."

The "me vale madre" mantra is a form of self-care and an emotional boundary that protects you from taking in people's shame and projections. Repeat it until you truly do not give a fuck about what people are saying about you because you are busy loving yourself and breaking generational cycles of self-silencing and abandonment. You are busy becoming a Badass Bonita.

According to Nedra Glover Tawwab, relationship expert, licensed therapist, and author of *Set Boundaries, Find Peace: A Guide to Reclaiming Yourself,* there are three types of boundary-setting styles. Tawwab shares how healthy boundaries require awareness of our own emotional, physical, and mental capacity in the moment in order to be able to communicate our needs clearly and effectively.[1] Healthy boundaries create interactions in which our past doesn't take up harmful space in our present nor does our anxiety for the future create rigid interactions. I believe that healthy boundaries require you to listen to yourself and respond accordingly. If your body is telling you it is hungry, you feed it. If your heart is telling you it feels unsafe, you listen to it. Perhaps your nervous system becomes activated when your partner screams at you. It may trigger a trauma response of when your caregivers used to scream at each other. You can communicate that to your partner. You can set a communication boundary that will provide you with more emotional safety during times of conflict. You can calmly and clearly let your partner know that you would like them to communicate in a respectful manner without yelling or cursing. This will not only teach them how to communicate with you in a way that feels loving to you, but it will also deepen your trust and help you build a secure attachment with yourself as you practice attuning to your own needs. This is part of your process of becoming a safe and loving person to yourself. Furthermore, this will help others be a safe and loving person to you. You show others how to love you by how well you love yourself.

HEALTHY BOUNDARIES

You know you are setting and upholding healthy boundaries when you are able to clearly and effectively communicate your needs. Not only do you say what you need and want, but you also take action in order to uphold the boundary. These two elements are essential to healthy boundary setting. It requires an intentional awareness of your emotional, mental, and physical capacities. You must know what you need, want, and what your capacity is in order to let others know.

Healthy boundaries look and feel like:

- Clear and effective communication.
- Listening to yourself and valuing your own voice.
- Saying no without apologizing or feeling guilty (trust your "No").
- Accepting other people's "No" without making them feel guilty or taking it personally.
- Cumpliendo tu palabra (keeping your word).
- Flexibility and honesty with your capacity and expectations.
- Awareness and comfort being vulnerable with others when it is appropriate and you've developed a trusting relationship.

Examples of healthy boundaries include:

- "I won't be able to help because I do not have the capacity at the moment. Thank you for understanding."
- "When we disagree on something, I need you not to yell at me. I may have to remove myself from this space and

come back when you are able to speak in a less aggressive tone."

- "Sí, puedo prestarte ese dinero. Necesito que me lo regreses en dos semanas."

After an extremely challenging and dramatic summer with my family, I was glad to hop on a plane back to Ithaca to start my junior year of college. My whole family came to drop me off. We embraced and cried. Then, I was surprised by the relief I felt when we got to the "Ticket Required Beyond this Point" sign. It was because none of them had a ticket besides me and they could no longer get to me once I crossed that point. I realized it was my parents I needed relief from.

It was then that I realized what boundaries felt like. It was boundaries that I needed, not plane tickets. The airport taught me a lot about boundaries to ensure safety and effective communication of said boundaries. There were signs everywhere which tell us where to go, how to properly walk through security, how to stand in the metal detector machine, what we are allowed to bring in, what we absolutely cannot carry with us, when to show up or we miss the flight, etc. Generally speaking, thanks to these boundaries there was a relative order we all followed. We know what to expect and we also know to expect consequences if we do not adhere to the airport safety guidelines. I began seeing my boundaries not as something selfish or wrong or mamona, but as the guidelines that would provide me with safety, relief, and a sense of agency over who enters my life, how they show up, and what they are allowed to bring with them.

RIGID BOUNDARIES

Rigid boundaries often feel like impenetrable walls people build around themselves in order to protect themselves. Rigid boundaries create distance as a protective mechanism. This boundary-setting style is an unhealthy way of keeping yourself safe. It stems from a fear of vulnerability and hyper-independence. Hyper-independence typically presents itself as a trauma response. Perhaps you were neglected as a child and learned not to depend on anyone but yourself. You developed a deep mistrust for others and expected everyone to disappoint you. If people didn't show up for you in the way that you needed them to, you may have learned to not let anyone show up for you now out of fear of rejection or disappointment. There may have been people who took advantage of you and therefore, you learned to doubt everyone's intentions and prefer to distance yourself just to be safe.

This type of boundary-setting style is a manifestation of an attachment wound typically seen in people with avoidant attachment style. For these individuals, distance feels safer, and closeness feels more dangerous, so they put systems in place in order to maintain the distance. Those with rigid boundaries rarely, if ever, change their boundaries. It is as if they built a fort around themselves and changing a boundary can feel like a breach in the fort. This must be avoided at all costs.

Rigid boundaries look like:

- Avoiding vulnerability and putting systems in place to prevent people from getting too close.
- Creating boundaries so people do not become needy or dependent on them and they don't depend on others.

- Building walls (emotionally, financially, physically).
- Not sharing (possessions, emotions, ideas).
- Cutting people off, blocking people.
- Treating boundaries like unbreakable rules that must be enforced at all costs.
- Saying no every time someone asks them for something because they don't want people to expect things from them.

Examples of rigid boundaries:

- "I never offer to help people because then they will always expect me to help them."
- "My rule is that no one can come over my house. No exceptions."

POROUS BOUNDARIES

If rigid boundaries are walls to a fort, porous boundaries are like papel picado, a traditional Mexican paper that's cut out with a similar technique as tissue paper snowflakes. Things can get in and out easily. They are not strong, nor do they provide much safety. These types of boundaries are usually nonexistent, barely there, or not enforced. You know you have this type of boundary-setting style if you feel guilty, overwhelmed, and like you are running on empty most of the time. There is a feeling of being out of control and chaotic. Your relationships do not feel stable nor reciprocal. You often tend to be the person that says yes to everything and everyone because you feel the need to please people in order to feel like they love you and accept you. You are terrified of disappointing people. Therefore, you never say no. You say yes even when you don't want to.

Overtime, you may feel a little resentful that you do everything for everyone, and people don't recognize all you do, or they take you for granted. You abandon your self-care, routines, needs, and dreams in order to show up for your family, friends, partner, or job. People often expect you to do things for them, praise you for how selfless you are, and may become dependent on you. You crave their approval, so you keep doing all the things they expect from you. You are not able to communicate your needs in an effective manner because oftentimes you don't know what they are or don't consider them important enough to say something. You tend to want to avoid conflict and silence yourself.

More times than not, people with anxious attachment tend to have a porous boundary-setting style. They believe that setting boundaries will create a distance or disappointment that will ruin the closeness they so desperately crave. Boundaries become a threat to the closeness that makes them something dangerous to those with anxious attachment. So, you would rather sacrifice your own wants and needs than disappoint those around you by putting up boundaries or speaking up for yourself.

Porous boundaries look like:

- Depending on others and/or having others depend on you.
- Inappropriate sharing.
- Enmeshment, or having no separation between you and others. Emotionally, their problems become your problems, you forget who you are as an individual without them.

- People pleasing.
- Fear of rejection.
- Staying in abusive, unsafe, unhealthy relationships out of fear of being alone.
- Tolerating mistreatment and/or disrespect.

Examples of porous boundaries:

- "Yes, I will work the double shift even though I had already told you I had a previous engagement. I'll make it work."
- "No, it's fine. I'm fine. Everything is fine. I'll take care of it, so you don't have to worry about anything."

Boundaries are essential to your becoming, mujer. Son parte de tu poder. Son arte. Son amor. Retoma tu poder. You gave it so freely to everyone else. They wanted you to be empty because they know how powerful you are when you are full. Eso los hace temblar. This is the part of your life where you realize you have the power to decide the rest of your life. It is how you teach others how to love you by how well you love yourself. It is a form of establishing safety for yourself and those around you.

You have the pen and the paper to write the rest of your story: plot, characters, finale. You are the artist, and this is your masterpiece. Escoge los colores con los que quieres pintar el resto de tu vida. They are the tools you use to piece yourself back together and unearth that inner guerrera. You are becoming a being who loves themselves fiercely, deeply, and wholeheartedly. Eres una guerrera que está lista y dispuesta para luchar por ella misma y ganar.

Porque por fin entendiste que vales la pena. You are worth fighting for. Boundaries are you establishing safety. Tú haciéndote cargo de ti misma. You are practicing self-love. Boundaries are you deciding you deserve peace instead of chaos, clarity instead of confusion, and agency instead of dependency.

Afirmaciones

I will take a deep breath and baby steps. It is okay for me to take my time and let me feel my feelings. I will give myself the opportunity to face my fears. I will be generous with how I love myself and others.

> *Respiraré profundo y daré pasitos. Me tomaré mi tiempo y me dejaré sentir mis sentimientos. Me daré la oportunidad de enfrentar mis miedos. Seré generosa con la manera en que me amo a mí y a otros.*

I will not forget my standards and I will hold my head high.

> *No me olvidaré de mis estándares. Mantendré mi mirada en alto.*

Boundaries, self-love, and confidence are part of my tools for liberation. I will use them to love, protect, and set myself free.

> *Mis límites, amor propio, y seguridad son parte de mis herramientas para mi liberación. Las utilizaré para amarme, protegerme y liberarme.*

My "No" is sufficient. It is necessary. Saying no does not make me selfish. I am saying yes to myself. This is part of my revolution.

Mi "no" es suficiente. Es necesario. Decir no, no me hace mala persona. Me estoy diciendo sí a mí misma. Esto es parte de mi revolución.

Chapter 11

Fuck Being Calladita

I grew up believing que calladita me veo más bonita.

Now I see it was another way I was oppressing and silencing myself.

Now whenever I hear "Calladita te ves más bonita," I say "Fuck that."

It breaks my heart how oftentimes this lie is passed down from one woman to another. Women shaming other women and themselves into silence—a tragedy and a reality. Audre Lorde, a Black lesbian poet and activist wrote about her experiences with self-silencing. A cancer diagnosis made her realize the urgency of her voice and the futility of her silence. She writes, "In becoming forcibly and essentially aware of my mortality, of what I wished and wanted from this life, however short it might be, priorities and omissions became strongly etched in a merciless light and what I most regretted were my silences." There are so many things we stop ourselves from saying due to shame and fear. Lorde goes on to say that our silence does not

protect us. This is true. My silence did not protect me. It only pro-
tected my oppressors. The shame their abuse and oppression put on
my shoulders did not protect me. My voice is what set me free. My
voice that I was so scared of was the key to my liberation. The shame
and silence I'd made my protectors were my main oppressors. Lorde
shares, "Of course I am afraid, because the transformation of silence
into language and action is an act of self-revelation, and that always
seems fraught with danger." Moving from a place of self-silencing to
a place of self-revelation is an act of revolutionary self-love. You are
believing in the value and power of your voice. You take action and
break your silence and turn it into liberation. Not only your own,
but for women around you. Healing and liberation always have a rip-
ple effect. It starts with you and heals generations. This is the beauty
and power of intergenerational healing. It is already alive within you.
Tus ancestres te están respaldando and the future generations are
thanking you for the courage to use your voice. So, instead of being a
woman that shames other women into silence, you are a woman who
uses her voice to love and liberate herself and other women. When
you speak up for yourself, you are speaking up for the many mujeres
who stayed quiet. By breaking the silence, you also break open a door
for other women to use their voice.

Audre Lorde's daughter once told her, "You're never really a
whole person if you remain silent, because there's always that one
little piece inside you that wants to be spoken out, and if you keep
ignoring it, it gets madder and hotter and hotter and if you don't
speak it out one day it will just jump up and punch you in the mouth
from the inside." This is true. I believe we were given a voice for a
reason. Our stories are ours for a reason. Our truth will yell at us
behind the silence we are hiding it under. It will come out one way
or another. Our healing asks us to stop being calladita. We must use

our voice in order to become whole. It is time to unsubscribe from shame and self-silencing.

It is time to subscribe to the Fuck Being Calladita lifestyle.

The Fuck Being Calladita lifestyle is a new way of being. In it, you actively use your voice as a tool for revolutionary self-love and collective liberation. My voice and my words changed my whole life. They were the catalysts and the energy that propelled my metamorphosis and evolution. The silence would've consumed me and killed me softly. This I know. ¡Tu voz es tu poder, mujer!

The FBC lifestyle is for those who are tired of silencing themselves and are ready to become a revolution. It is not a one-size-fits-all. You get to say fuck that or fuck yes to whatever feels most loving to you. Say fuck yes first to yourself. Say fuck that to whatever feels oppressive, keeps you from growing, or causes you harm. Then say fuck yes to anything or anyone who adds to your light, helps you heal and expand, and helps you love yourself better. You get to choose. It is not another set of rules. Better yet, it is an invitation to say fuck that to all the rules you were taught. Fuck yes to choosing how you want to live, what you want to say, and who you want to be.

From the moment I spoke up about being abused, my life was never the same. This was the beginning of my Fuck Being Calladita lifestyle. I just didn't know it. Initially, there was resistance. There usually is. No te preocupes. When one part of a system changes, the whole system has to change. Naturally, as humans we resist change, especially if it asks us to dismantle existing systems of oppression. The ones who resist the most are the ones who benefit from these systems the most. Se tenía que decir y se dijo. The people around me resisted and tried to shame me back into silence. I resisted their resistance. They fought and gave me the silent treatment. I suffered, yet I didn't go back to the old way. Once they saw I was not going to remain quiet, they had to take time and evaluate what to do with me—la que ya no se queda callada.

Slowly, they started to reintegrate me back. However, pretty soon they realized it wasn't me reintegrating into their system. It was them integrating into mine. I had jumped off their sinking ship and built my own while they were busy shutting me out. In my ship, there were boundaries, there was no shame, no one was expected to stay quiet about things that mattered to them, and most importantly, there was love—real, nonabusive love. These were uncharted territories for all of us. At times, I could feel they were grateful. Other times, I was sure they hated me. They hated talking about feelings. They shamed me for wanting to talk about the past. They hated talking about the abuse, machismo, therapy, and boundaries. It made them extremely uncomfortable.

There was a power within me that knew I could not go back to being a calladita. I was doing this for the women before me who had no choice but to callarse. Silence was their destination, and they knew it almost from the moment they were born. I am doing it for the women and niñas who come after me. I do not want them to go through the same battles, the silence, the shame, the shutout, and the absolute bullshit I had to deal with when I first started using my voice. My prayer for the next generation is that the Fuck Being Calladita lifestyle is one they are born into, not one they have to cry, claw, and crawl into like I did.

Once you say yes to the FBC lifestyle, your life will never be the same. Es como si alguien prendiera un fuego en tu garganta y no lo quisieras apagar. Más bien, abres tu boca para que salga. It is as if someone lights a fire in your throat and you do not want to extinguish it. Better yet, you open your throat, so it roars out of you. When you open your mouth, it will consume the chains, the silence, the patriarchy, the oppression, the shame which used to consume you. Así que abre la boca, y ruge, mujer.

The Fuck Being Calladita lifestyle invites you to share your story and speak your truth. It does not mean hablar a lo menso or speaking words that will cause harm. FBC is realizing your voice has power to heal and liberate. Tu voz es medicina. Use it with intention, purpose, y sobre todo con mucho, mucho amor. Your voice is an instrument of love and liberation. When they told us, "Calladita te ves más bonita" they made us believe our voice (if used) was more of a weapon we had to be afraid of. Fuck that—our voice is medicine. When we get tired of being calladitas, that's when the revolution begins.

Badass Bonita, if you are ready to subscribe to the Fuck Being Calladita lifestyle, repeat after me:

- Calladita te ves más bonita. Fuck that.
- Las guapas se aguantan. Fuck that.
- Women should submit to their husbands. Fuck that.
- Women shouldn't speak up at church. Fuck that.
- Women belong in the kitchen. Fuck that.
- Women should stay at home and watch the kids. Fuck that.
- You shouldn't wear that because men can't control themselves. Fuck that.
- Si te trata mal es porque le gustas. Fuck that.
- Behind every good man is a good woman. Fuck that.
- Boys will be boys. Fuck that.
- She's asking for it. Fuck that.
- Silencing ourselves. Fuck that.
- Protecting abusers and oppressors. Fuck that.
- Not holding men accountable. Fuck that.
- Not going to therapy or healing. Fuck that.

- Believing our needs aren't important. Fuck that.
- Believing our opinions aren't important. Fuck that.
- Upholding machista values. Fuck that.
- Letting our past dictate our future. Fuck that.
- Upholding the belief women are only meant to serve others. Fuck that.
- Letting our past determine our future. Fuck that.
- Repeating toxic cycles of abuse, shame, and silence. Fuck that.
- Being ashamed of who we are. Fuck that.
- Hiding and/or shrinking ourselves. Fuck that.
- Aguantar pendejadas. Fuck that.
- People-pleasing. Fuck that.
- Punishing our bodies for what other people did. Fuck that.
- Believing we are not worthy of love. Fuck that.
- Conforming to society's beauty standards. Fuck that.
- Conforming to the gender norms and binary system. Fuck that.
- El qué dirán. Fuck that.
- Trying to be perfect. Fuck that.
- Talking shit about ourselves or other women. Fuck that.
- Fixing another queen's crown. Fuck yes.
- Saying, "Me vale." Fuck yes.
- Doing what we want because we want to do it. Fuck yes.
- Not asking for permission to be ourselves. Fuck yes.
- Embracing our imperfections. Fuck yes.
- Embracing our queerness. Fuck yes.
- Being a bad bitch with a soft heart. Fuck yes.
- Forgiving ourselves. Fuck yes.

- Setting boundaries. Fuck yes.
- "No me voy a dejar." Fuck yes.
- Speaking up for ourselves and trusting the power of our voices. Fuck yes.
- Sharing our truths and stories. Fuck yes.
- Unsubscribing from shame. Fuck yes.
- Going to therapy. Fuck yes.
- Trusting our timing and the nonlinear ways of our healing journey. Fuck yes.
- Choosing to love ourselves un poquito más cada día. Fuck yes.
- Believing that being vulnerable is not a weakness. Fuck yes.
- Letting ourselves feel our feelings. Fuck yes.
- Knowing our worth and acting accordingly. Fuck yes.
- Knowing we are healing generational trauma. Fuck yes.
- Knowing our existence is a beautiful resistance and a work of art. Fuck yes.

The Fuck Being Calladita lifestyle es para las que ya se cansaron de estar calladitas y están listas para convertirse en una revolución.

Unsubscribing from shame and subscribing to the "Fuck Being Calladita" lifestyle is a journey you don't have to walk alone. You need support when you're fighting shame, much like you need light to see in the darkness. Surround yourself with people who will help you fight your shame by loving you well. Surround yourself with people who will say fuck yes every time you use your voice. Find the people who will celebrate you speaking up for yourself rather than shame you. Find the ones who will love how much you love yourself—the ones who will want you to heal and shine once more. Surround yourself with art. Create art. Become art. Have those difficult conversations con tus tías criticonas. Hold men accountable. Hold yourself close. Set those boundaries. Join a support group. Hold your head high. Use your voice even if it trembles. Raise your hand in class. Realize your voice can change lives. Say, "Fuck that!" to all who try to silence you. Take your ass to therapy. And please: fuck being calladita.

> Reflect on your relationship with shame. What are the stories shame tells you about yourself? What are the ways in which shame has stopped you or kept you from going after what you want? Once you explore when your relationship with shame began and identify the toxic patterns you experience with shame, I invite you to write shame a break-up letter in which you unsubscribe from it.

Afirmaciones

I will speak, fight for, and commit to my dreams.
> *Yo usaré mi voz, lucharé y me comprometeré a realizar mis sueños.*

My silence does not equal my beauty. I will no longer silence myself.
> *Mi belleza no está vinculada a mi silencio. Ya no me voy a callar.*

I am beginning and becoming a revolution.
> *Estoy iniciando y convirtiéndome en una revolución.*

My voice can change lives, starting with mine.
Mi voz puede cambiar vidas, incluyendo la mía.

I will use my voice to state my needs even when it terrifies me, I have not fought so hard to feel so small again. My past, present, and future will thank me.
Usaré mi voz para comunicar mis necesidades aunque tenga miedo. No he luchado tanto para sentirme tan pequeña otra vez. Mi pasado, presente y futuro me lo agradecerán.

Chapter 12

The Mariposa Effect

Y̶ou are an active participant in the intergenerational healing and collective liberation of your people—our people. The way you love yourself is directly connected to the collective's liberation. The words you speak and the messages you pass on will impact generations to come. Eres poderosa, mujer. How will you use your voice to usher in liberation, healing, and strength? What messages are you uprooting? What cycles will stop with you? What messages are you planting like seeds in your garden? Breathe in and acknowledge the strength within you. Eres luz. Eres una guerrera. Eres una Badass Bonita. There is revolutionary love running through your veins.

One of the women that inspired me to fly was Frida Kahlo. She was the first woman I read that told me she had wings. "Feet, what do I need you for when I have wings to fly?"

I remember thinking this was revolutionary: a woman with wings. A woman who can fly. I want to be that. How do I become that? I began studying the life of Frida Kahlo to see if it was possible for me to one day have wings to fly as well. Her declaration of her wings and freedom ignited a fire in me to get my own. This woman didn't magically get her wings and fly happily ever after. She wove them together with her tears, paint, blood, and sorrow. All of those were ingredients also present in my life. Perhaps, I too could transform them into something that would help me fly. I love how she spoke her mind and called out the gringos for their privilege, classism, and racism. I loved that she loved women.

I lived in the same neighborhood in Coyoacán that Frida Kahlo grew up in. My home was a couple of blocks from her Casa Azul. Mine was orange. Even now, I cannot fathom a woman walking around the streets of Coyoacán in a man's suit. Imagine her doing that in 1924! Tremenda. Una mujer que se atrevió a ser ella misma. Aun con sus imperfecciones, ella se amó y se aceptó. No fingió ser perfecta, ni intentó ser lo que la sociedad esperaba de ella. Una mujer salvaje pintando, llorando y resistiendo por las calles de Coyoacán. Ahora sus pinturas están por todo el mundo. Y sus alas nos han dado a muchas permiso para encontrar las nuestras y volar.

One of the things about Frida that gave my queer girl's corazón wings was her love affair with one of my heroes: Chavela Vargas, a lesbiana, Mexicana born in Costa Rica who became one of the most influential singers and queer icons of her time. She was notorious for dressing "como un hombre," singing in her deep, penetrating voice, and breaking a number of cultural norms. For them to be two queer mujeres en México, not hiding their queerness, gave queer women across generations wings. After decades of people inquiring about her sexual identity, Chavela Vargas responded, "I had to fight to be me and get respect, and to carry that stigma, for me, is pride. Carrying the label of lesbian. I am not bragging, I'm not preaching, but I don't deny it. I had to face society and the Church, which condemn gay people. It's absurd. How do you judge someone who has been born this way?"[1] Each one of those words comes from the heart of someone que se atrevió a ser libre y a la cual la sociedad la llamó loca. Pero esa libertad que ella misma se dio, nadie se la pudo quitar. Y esa libertad me acercó a la mía. This is the Mariposa Effect.

The Mariposa Effect happens when one woman gives herself wings and inspires other women to do the same. It is a manifestation of collective liberation. This is a movement founded on love—for oneself and for the collective. When I choose to love myself, I am choosing to love myself enough to heal, and I know that when I heal, my healing will have a ripple effect. Our healing is part of a movement of liberation. It is not an isolated act. Revolution and liberation are ways of living, breathing, and thinking. I do not think we are ever truly done. We have to be aware enough to be constantly setting ourselves free from oppression, shame, and fear. It is a constant state of change, a metamorphosis toward our wings. We need different sets of wings to carry us through different seasons. We need each other too. When it comes to collective liberation, we must be acutely aware of how much we need one another to give ourselves wings. There are systems in place to oppress us. There are people in place to liberate us. We are those people.

We are those wild women teaching other women to be wild. We are those wild women creating medicine and leaving it everywhere we go for others to find and heal their wounds. We are those wild women weaving together bandages with our tears to make other women's wounds stop bleeding. Nos cuidamos. Nos apapachamos. Nos escuchamos. Nos damos fuerzas. Nos liberamos. We care for one another. We hold one another. We listen to one another. We give each other strength. We set ourselves free. We help each other heal. Collective liberation is less about how much we fight for one another and more about how well we love one another. How well we love one another greatly depends on how well we love ourselves.

It is all connected.

It is the Mariposa Effect.

The forerunners of this Mariposa Effect have been Black and trans women. They are often the most oppressed and the ones who have set the most people free. Black and trans women have been a constant example of human beings giving themselves wings and liberating themselves because no one else has fought for them the way they have fought for themselves. They are, as Paulo Freire puts it, "an example in the struggle for their redemption"—teachers in the art of setting themselves free. Those who have had to fight for their freedom know what it is like to be enslaved. They have greater compassion when they see others still in slavery. Those are the ones most likely to break the chains of their hermanas. This is love in action: the love that makes you set your hermanas free because you know the suffering caused by living in chains. Assata Shakur shares, "People get used to anything. The less you think about your oppression, the more your tolerance for it grows. After a while, people just think oppression is the normal state of things. But to become free, you have to be acutely aware of being a slave." It is this awareness that puts the fire within us to seek our freedom. It is love that sets us free. It is this awareness that helps us notice when our hermanas are suffering. It is love that drives us to set us all free.

It is a state of being in which we want to see us all with wings. Quiero que llenemos el cielo con nuestras alas y en el piso dejemos atrás las cadenas que nos ataban. I want us to fill the sky with the colors of our wings and leave the chains that once tied us laying on the ground.

Revolution and liberation are ways of living, breathing, and thinking. I do not think we are ever truly done. We have to be aware enough to be constantly setting ourselves free from oppression, shame, and fear. Shakur reminds us that revolution is about change and that the first place change begins is in ourselves.

There was a moment when I realized that the messages that I will pass on to the next generation have to be messages of love and liberation. Yo no iba a pasar los mensajes que me habían pasado a mí como veneno que todavía ardía y me encadenaba. I refused to pass down the messages that were passed down to me like venom that still burned in my throat and wrapped itself around me like chains. I couldn't sit still, because I felt this moment required action. It required me to do something in order to seal this commitment and decision. The reason we've passed down so much pain and trauma is not because our mamis had the evil intention to ruin our lives and set us up for years of therapy. It was simply because they were busy trying to survive. They were not aware of the messages they were passing on. Part of the problem is passivity. We get accustomed to accepting things as they are even though they are causing us to bleed. We learn to tolerate abuse and mistreatment. We accept the unacceptable. We continue the cycle without consciousness. Revolution requires change.

In that moment of realization, I grabbed the most powerful weapons I had: paper and pen. I began writing down the messages I wish I had heard growing up and the ones I was going to pass down. I read them out loud to myself. I felt the healing power of these words. They were new words written and spoken with love and with the intention of bringing in healing. There's a difference when we set intention to our words and are aware of the messages we are passing forward.

The first time I read this letter out loud to anyone other than myself was at the We All Grow Latina summit. The room was full with about six hundred vibrant, buzzing Latinas. The energy was palpable and invigorating. I was wearing a bright, red sequined dress. The style was a mix of something Selena and Paquita la del Barrio might wear. I had gotten it for forty dollars at Ross and didn't care that the invitation had said semi-casual. This floor-length sequin gown was coming on that stage with me. I stepped onto the stage and took a deep breath. People have described my performances as stand-up poetry. Soy una payasa. I like making people laugh while sharing poems, stories, and chismes with them. The atmosphere changed when I introduced the "Mija letter." I let them know why I wrote it and who I wrote it for. An expectant silence filled the room. My voice was soft, yet strong. A quiet power anchored me.

Mija,
I want to show you my world, mi cultura, nuestra cultura.
Nuestra comida y nuestras canciones. Our beautiful español.
Quiero que conozcas el amor: to love and not be afraid of lov-
ing. Whoever you choose to love. I want you to feel safe, worthy,
confident enough to receive love the way you deserve to be loved.
I want you to know that I will always choose you first—no
man, struggle, or anything in this world can come between us.
Absolutamente nada, mija.
*   Mija, I was created to love and protect you. I will give my*
life up for you. You are my child, mija.
*   Made from my heart, blood, soul, body—yet you are your*
own person. I also love that about you. God trusted me enough
to love you and raise you. This world is blessed to have you.

Mija, be kind. Keep your mind and heart open so fear doesn't come in. Mija, eres hermosa in every way. You are beautiful. Mija, eres fuerte. You can do all things. You have a stubborn-ass mama and all of heaven cheering you on. Mija, be the kind of human that loves well. In order to do this, you must first learn to love yourself. I hope I love myself well enough that you can learn from me how to love you. Then, you can love others freely and fully. If someone is hungry, feed them. If someone is naked, clothe them. If someone is lonely, hold them. You will always have enough. You will always be more than enough. Mija, be brave. Courage and resilience runs in our veins. Nuestros ancestors were warriors, ¡los más valientes! Siempre le echaron ganas. They taught us: "¡Sí se puede!" Mija, we come from Aztec blood, mighty warriors, lovers, and protectors. Mija, we are seeds, nopales, mariposas valientes y resistentes. Mija, grow and love and love and grow. Do not be afraid to be beautiful. Do not be afraid to shine. Mija, I promise to love you with unconditional, never-ending love. Mija, I promise I will mess up, make mistakes, and never, ever be perfect. Mija, I promise I will learn, keep trying, and never ever give up. Mija, I promise to love you for who you are and not for who you "should" be. Mija, life isn't perfect or always pretty, but it is beautiful and worth living it with all we've got. I will be there with you every step of the way. Mija, I will show you Love through my life and actions. Love will show itself to you.

You are glorious.
Eres tuya.

When I was done, all I could hear was sniffles and mocos. I looked around and everyone was crying. They were wiping their eyes with the napkins on their tables. Eyeliner was running down some of their cheeks. Once I got off the stage, so many women came up to me.

"That letter healed parts of me I didn't know were still hurting."

"You said everything I wanted to hear as a little girl."

"Mi mami se murió, pero dijiste cosas que ella me decía y necesitaba escuchar otra vez."

"I'm going to read it to my daughter."

"I'm going to read it to my mom because she needed to hear those words too."

"Gracias, mija."

Those interactions taught me how much these messages matter and how much words can heal us and bring us together. Their hands were reaching out to me and touching my heart, much like the hands from the vision with Botánica Melo, a mother–daughter healing duo who offer traditional healing practices. The daughter is a singer, sound healer, and photographer with a profound, powerful, and soft soul. The mother is a fierce, gentle, wise therapist, sanadora, and guide. Nuestras palabras son las gotas de lluvia que caen y riegan las semillas plantadas en el jardín. Our words are the drops of rain that water the seeds planted in our garden.

I want you to write a similar letter full of all the things you needed to hear as a niña growing up and all the things you wish to pass on to the next generation. Read it out loud to yourself. And if you ever get the chance to read it on a stage, do it. You don't know how many wounded hearts your words will bring medicine to.

THE SPIRAL OF HEALING

One of the most beautiful realizations of what intergenerational healing and the mariposa effect feels like happened during a healing ceremony with Botánica Melo. I want to share it with you and invite you to do a similar visualization. When I walked into the room, they had it set up beautifully. There were candles and flowers arranged in a spiral on the floor. The daughter was sitting on the floor with her drum. The mother welcomed me and asked me to lay down as she set a blanket on top of the flowers on the floor. She then wrapped the blanket around me as if I was in a cocoon. I closed my eyes. I felt safe. Then they started to sing over me. The daughter sang while the mother led me in a visualization.

At first, I saw myself laying there as I was. Then I felt a warmth in my heart. It came from the hands of the women in my family. I could see these hands with all the shades of brown surround my heart. They were blessing me and giving me strength. They were also saying thank you. This surprised me because I was convinced the women in my family were going to hate me, o que me iban a regañar, since I do a lot of the things they told me I shouldn't. Yet they surprised me by saying thank you. I felt tears sliding down my cheeks. Then, they said, "Mija, tú eres una guerrera. Es el momento de levantarte. Sigue adelante. Estamos contigo."

The mother's voice whispered, "Picture yourself walking into a field toward a mountain. When you get to the top, you will find someone waiting for you."

It was my inner niña.

My first response was to hold her. I sat there and held her. Then, I felt my mom come from behind me and hold both me and my inner niña. Then, my grandma came and held us. Then my great-grandma and her mami and her mami and so on and so forth. My inner niña felt safe being held by all these women in her life. She felt happy. I thought, "This is what intergenerational healing feels like." I'd always just wanted to be held by these women without shame. It felt like pure love running from one generation to the next.

Then the visual expanded to an aerial view of this scene of women holding each other. It looked like a spiral with my inner niña at the center and the older generations on the outer parts of the spiral. All of a sudden, it shifted. My ancestors told me: "You know what it's like to be held and loved. Now it is time to for you to open your wings." The oldest women who were on the outer parts of the spiral then shifted toward the center while each younger generation expanded a little at a time toward the outer parts. The spiral kept getting bigger. At first, I didn't understand why this shift was happening. Then they told me:

> *Your grandmother started to think about new possibilities that your great-grandmother couldn't even imagine.*
> *What your grandmother silenced, your mother started to whisper.*
> *What your mami whispered, you started to speak out loud.*
> *Your daughters are going to yell it.*
> *Their daughters are going to sing it.*
> *Their daughters are going to dance it.*
> *It will keep expanding.*
> *We will keep expanding.*

In this picture, I went from being this little niña being held in the center to being the next generation, on the outside of the spiral with my arms spread open and my heart laid bare. I was leading the way with my heart, my voice, my mind, and my eyes open toward the next generation. I felt a responsibility and honor saying, doing, being what they needed, but couldn't. They were thanking me and loving me for being what they couldn't imagine they could be. They thanked me for speaking what they thought they'd have to live their whole lives silencing.

What do you do with this freedom you've given to yourself? You learn to live instead of surviving. You learn to dance with yourself at night. You give yourself pleasure. You get angry. You dismantle systems of oppression. You connect. You make art. You make love. You create. You destroy. You give birth to new beginnings. You realize that this freedom—this wilderness returns you to the essence of you. It's always been there. It leads you to the clearing in the forest in which you can ask your soul: "What do you want?"

"Quiero seguir siendo libre."

If you were born into trauma, oppression, and darkness, your soul knows what it is like not to be free. Survival isn't freedom. When you give your soul a taste of freedom, it will do everything in its power to not go back. You can't go back. You have the strength of your ancestors holding you up so that you can continue your path toward liberation. It is a movement forward, one step at a time, agarradas de las manos con las mujeres que vinieron antes y las que vienen después. Somos una trenza de libertad: las de antes, las de ahorita y las que vendrán: nos necesitamos, y juntas nos hacemos más fuertes.

We need to usher in liberation into all the parts of our lives in which we do not feel free or in which we aren't growing. Our process of liberation must take into consideration institutional systems of oppression, family systems, relationships, and internalized oppression. There are times we must set ourselves free from thoughts infused with shame, fear, and self-hate. There are other times we must set ourselves free from the cycles of abuse and neglect present in our families. There are times we must set ourselves free from relationships that are slowly taking away our agency and will to live. There are times when we must dismantle entire systems of oppression in schools, court systems, and immigrant detention centers that are threatening reproductive rights and trans lives. We need to seek out liberation and marry ourselves to the revolution.

I divorced the white man and married the revolution.
I committed to liberation.
I got a restraining order against machismo.
I said "I do" to women getting their wings.
I vow to be a reason that this world is better for our children and our children's children.
I vow to not believe my beauty is tied to my silence.
Prometo no quedarme calladita or pass on the lie que calladita me veo más bonita.
My beauty is tied to my power and how well I've learned to love myself—this is the genesis of my own revolution.
I fell in love with you, revolución.
You taught me the power within me.
El poder de mi voz, mis palabras, mi cuerpo y mi corazón.
The power of my voice, my words, my body, and my heart.
Revolución, I will walk beside you.
I will get to know you and learn from you.
Revolution: we are one. You and I. I am you and you are me.
Te amo porque me amo.
I love you because I love me.
Me amas porque me amo.
You love me because I love me.

Somos porque nos necesitamos.
We are because we need each other.
Sin ti no soy y sin mí no eres.
I cannot exist without you nor you without me.
Somos.
Me uno contigo, revolución amada.
I join myself to you, beloved revolution.

Your soul will tell you when it is not connected. Your soul will tell you when it needs more of you and less of someone else. Your soul will let you know when it is not feeling free. Escucha.

I pass this message on to you: the love you give yourself and the love you give to this world is the love that is needed to give us all wings.

Mujer, your voice is an instrument of love for collective liberation and intergenerational healing. Do not ever silence yourself again.

Nunca más te quedes calladita.

CONCLUSION

When a caterpillar's DNA is tested, it says: "butterfly." It may not start off as a butterfly or even look like a butterfly, but its entire molecular system is designed to transform into what it was created to become: a winged, beautiful creature.

Same goes with us.

You were born and created to become the most powerful, beautiful, liberated version of yourself. It is in your DNA. Freedom is the destiny that belongs to everyone. Society teaches us to wait for someone to give us permission to be free, even when we have the key. You have the key.

The goal of the work that you are doing is to learn to live the most peaceful and authentic life you could possibly live. This work is meant to be the bridge that helps you go from surviving to healing, and from healing to living. When you make the decision to cross that bridge, you are doing it not only for yourself, but for the generations before you that never made it to the edge. For your abuela that endured what she had to silently in order to survive. For your mami, who whispered her dreams in the dark to herself, wanting better for her mother and better for herself. Better for you. For yourself, who can now shout, who can now stand the fuck up for yourself and other women.

You are standing on this bridge of self-discovery with the tools to craft the future you want. One with intention, one with boundaries, one with self-awareness, one with ancestral wisdom, and one with love. It may feel uncomfortable to fully accept your position on this bridge. Everyone reaches a point in their journey when they come across discomfort, and I dare you to feel it. Embrace it with your whole self, because building the reality you want to exist in will be met with discomfort from deep inside yourself—or from people that are witnessing your growth. The peace that is waiting for you on the other side of that discomfort is worth it. I promise. You are worth that peace.

If you are at a point in your life in which you feel like you never got a chance, a break, a moment for yourself, let me be the one to tell you that this can be that moment. This can be the time when you choose whether to continue down the prewritten path for you or choose to change direction. If you are not ready for it now, that's okay. Approach this book and this journey again when you feel called to it. Any time is a good time to heal.

You are in the process of becoming a more badass, beautiful, healthy, powerful version of you. And through this process, you will pave the way and give permission for other mujeres to do the same. Metamorphosis is alchemy. It takes great power, magic, and love to transform from one being to another, from one version of yourself into the next.

Change is beautiful.

Change is badass.

And change starts with you.

You have all you need to give yourself wings.

Ahora, ¡atrévete a volar!

APPENDIX

Badass Bonita Manifesto

Your words, existence, and heart are medicina, Badass Bonita.
Tienes alas. You have wings.
Your voice is necessary and powerful.
Tu voz es poderosa y necesaria.
You have revolutionary self-love running through your veins.
Tienes amor revolucionario corriendo por tus venas.
You are an instrument of intergenerational healing.
Eres un instrumento de sanación intergeneracional.
It is time to unapologetically embrace the strength of who
you are and who you are becoming.
Eres libre, atrevida y loca.
You are a wild woman setting other wild women free.
You are magic and medicine.
Es hora de vivir sin miedo y con ganas.
Ya no eres calladita.
You are a mujer who uses her voice as an instrument of liberation.
You are an imperfect human being who loves herself.
You are a mujer who gave herself wings.
Eres una sinvergüenza.
You are shameless and free.
You are a Badass Bonita.

Badass Bonitas are whoever they choose to be.
We do whatever the fuck we want, because we know
who the fuck we are.
Badass Bonitas make this world more beautiful.
We give ourselves wings.
Llenamos los cielos con los colores de nuestras alas.
We honor where we come from and we know
where we are going: liberation.
Vivimos sin miedo y con ganas.
We fight for ourselves and for one another.
We don't let the world tell us who we are:
we tell the world who we are.
What we have to say matters because who we are matters.
Badass Bonitas break intergenerational curses and usher in
intergenerational healing.
Somos medicina salvaje. Somos magia.
Somos las semillas que decidieron luchar.
We set boundaries. We choose healing. We are love.
We are the baddest bitches, with the softest of hearts.
Badass Bonitas set one another free.
We look at each other con ojos de amor.
My wings will remind you of your own.
We are flowers. Together we are a garden. I want to see us blooming
y llenando el cielo con el color de nuestras alas.
Badass Bonitas love themselves—in a revolutionary way.
We move mountains and make this world more badass.
We dismantle systems of oppression.
We redefine what is beautiful.
We embrace queerness.
No nos dejamos.

Badass Bonitas somos y seremos.
Nos transformamos.
We are not afraid of our metamorphosis.
We evolve una y otra vez.
Abrazamos lo que nos libera.
Soltamos lo que nos oprime.
We live fully.
Sabemos lo que merecemos: amor y no chingaderas.
Sembramos semillas de amor.
We are loving ourselves into gardens.
Badass Bonitas: a collective of mujeres
sanando, amando y liberando.

You are a beautiful, wild, badass mujer.
Una mujer que se dio alas y no se dejó.
No te dejaste callar.
Más bien, te dejaste vivir, sanar y amar.
Te dejaste ser libre.
You let yourself heal and grow in peace.
You chose peace.
You chose yourself.
This is what being a Badass Bonita is all about.

Ser y dejar ser libre.

Affirmations para Badass Bonitas

There is power in your words, mujer. The words you speak over yourself and about yourself are a big part of your becoming. Speak words of love. May your words be medicine for your soul. May your words break cycles. May your words reframe thoughts and restructure neural pathways. Your words can and will change your life. Affirmations keep your becoming at the forefront of your mind. These affirmations are you co-creating with the universe and connecting with your essence. They are the pathway to your becoming.

Affirmations are most effective when you say them out loud, preferably looking at yourself in the mirror. Make them personal by inserting your name in the beginning or at the end. Perhaps your name or a loving nickname you have for yourself or your inner niña.

BADASS AFFIRMATIONS
PARA MUJERES

My life is a gift given to me daily. I will fill it with people and experiences that make me feel alive. I will live a life well lived.

> *Mi vida es un regalo que recibo todos los días. La llenaré de personas y experiencias que me hagan sentir viva. Voy a vivir una vida bien vivida.*

I am allowed to feel the full range of my emotions. I will be gentle with my heart as it learns how to feel. My heart is healing and blooming.

> *Me doy permiso de sentir todas mis emociones. Seré tierna con mi corazón mientras aprende a sentir. Mi corazón está sanando y floreciendo.*

My softness is part of my strength. My vulnerability shows the places I've healed and I am willing to let the light in.

> *Mi ternura es parte de mi fuerza. Mi vulnerabilidad destaca los lugares en los cuales he sanado y estoy dispuesta a dejar entrar a la luz.*

I am a bad bitch with a soft heart.

> *Soy una mujer chingona con un corazón tierno.*

Doing things just because I want to is a sufficient reason to do them. It is not wrong. It is not selfish. It is me listening to myself and taking action.

> *Hacer las cosas porque quiero es razón suficiente para hacerlas. No es malo. No es egoísta. Es una demostración de que me estoy escuchando y respondiendo a ello.*

I am in the process of getting my wings. I am in my metamorphosis: caterpillar, chrysalis, breakthrough, butterfly.

> *Estoy en proceso de recibir mis alas. Estoy en mi metamorfosis: gusano, capullo, transformación, mariposa.*

I will not abandon myself.

> *No me abandonaré.*

I will protect and fight for my dreams.
  Protegeré mis sueños y lucharé por ellos.

I am ready and capable of learning new things.
  Estoy lista y soy capaz de aprender cosas nuevas.

I love myself enough to not stay the same.
  Me amo lo suficiente para no quedarme igual.

I am decolonizing and fighting the patriarchy with my art, poetry, and existence.
  Estoy descolonizando y luchando contra el patriarcado con mi arte, mi poesía y mi existencia.

I resist by resting. My joy is resistance. My voice is revolutionary.
  Yo resisto cuando descanso. Mi alegría es resistencia. Mi voz es revolucionaria.

My imperfections make me human. I will let myself be human today.
  Mis imperfecciones me hacen humana. Hoy me dejaré ser humana.

I am generous and abundant. My people taught me how to make magic out of nothing.
  Soy generosa y abundante. Mi gente me enseñó a hacer magia de la nada.

My skin is beautiful. It is kissed by the sun. It is the color of the earth, the color of life.
  Mi piel es hermosa, besada por el sol. Es del color de la tierra, del color de la vida.

My body will always belong to me. I get to make all the rules.
Mi cuerpo es y siempre será mío. Yo pongo todas las
reglas.

Me and my people are not going anywhere but up. We are rising
as our roots grow deeper. I bless the next generation when I pass
down my cultura.
Yo y mi gente no nos vamos p'abajo, solo p'arriba. Nos
levantamos mientras nuestras raíces se profundizan.
Bendecimos a la próxima generación al pasarle nuestra
cultura.

As I rise, I bring others up with me. As I heal, I heal those that
came before me and will come after.
Al elevarme, ayudo a otros a elevarse conmigo. Al sanar,
ayudo a sanar a los que me precedieron y los que
vendrán después.

Add to this list and pass it on.

May your words become medicina for other Badass Bonitas.

AGRADECIMIENTOS

I want to start by thanking God for loving me the way They do. Thank you for those jasmine flowers on the bus stop on Ventura Boulevard. Thank you for the butterflies every time I sat beneath the orange tree to write and pray. Gracias por acompañarme a través de cada desierto, montaña, mar, tormenta, latido. Thank you for every word, tear, and miracle. This is for and with you.

Gracias a mi familia. Rach Gang, our counterparts Bs&Hs, and the bebés. I am forever grateful for all we have been through together and how each time we come out softer and stronger. Gracias a mi mami, que me dio luz y siempre me recordó, "Dios ha puesto el mundo en tus manos." Gracias a mi Tita, la Loba, que me dio tanto fuego y amor. Gracias por amarme a tu manera y ser mi cómplice y compañera en este camino. Gracias a mi Nina, tía Irene, Shuleira, Nere, Eny, mi abue, tía Chely y mi tío Pepe. Gracias a los Argueta for taking me in since I was little Kimberly. Thank you to my dad, bonus mom, Gen, Kyle, Grandma Rosa, Aunt Cindy, Nicole, and Savannah. *Grazie mille* a Rosalia y Marco Maddalena, *vi voglio bene. Bacino, bacino.* Thank you to my chosen family for taking me in and loving me deep. Gracias a Chancho por ser mi compañero y cómplice. Gracias por enseñarme, acompañarme y amarme tanto.

Gracias a todas las mujeres que me han acompañado en mi camino. Gracias a Ms. Sánchez, my first-grade teacher. She was that adult in my life who made the difference by believing in me. She taught me about the metamorphosis de las mariposas. It changed my life and inspired so much of this book. Gracias a Leonor; Ms. De La Torre; Ms. Bright; Ms. Álvarez; my drill team at Fair Avenue, who became my family when my family was falling apart; Mrs. Schroeder; Daniela; Nidia; my sista Pau (tbbsl); Hermana Lilian por recibirme como familia; Mrs. Drapkin; Kelly Cullen, my spiritual mama; Shauna-Kay; Nirel; Onica; Brenda; Sarah B. anamchara; Fatima, my ride or die; the women at Hope Place; Misty, for painting new colors in my life and taking us to the lavender fields; Tasha Black; K. Woo, Doris, por caminar conmigo; Raquel, for helping me in my first vending event; Maribel G.; my fairy godmother Ana Flores; la bichota Davi; Angélica María; Paula Duran and Rocío, my Pisces roomies; ASV; Doris in the desert; Mari and Krista, my queens; Nancy G.; Emma Rubí; Lizbeth Franco; Dany Pérez; Dani Manzur, nuestra madrina de Ocotlán; MJ, my sponsor; Frida y Chavela; my therapist, Flor, que me acompañó en mi lucha por mí; Dr. María, por el trabajo con mi niña interior; Dra. Mariel Buque for being an inspiration y acompañarme en este camino; Virginia for supporting me all these years and for the important and intentional work you do for our community; Botánica Melo; and that random lady on a Facebook forum who told me, "Your life is just as important."

I want to give a special thank you to Sharon Blake. God brought you into my life with such a beautiful purpose. If it was not for you, your courage, your story, and Life Chronicles Publishing, I would not be here today. You were the one who made me believe I was a writer. You brought *Mariposa* out into the world and changed my life forever. I will love and admire you always. You've changed so many lives just by being you.

Thank you to my badass book doula team. Hannah, this book wouldn't be here if it was not for your grace, apapachos, and guerrera spirit. You brought the fire and earth this book needed to flourish. You ran and walked and crawled this race with me and passed on the baton when you did all you could and gave all the love you gave. Nana, thank you for receiving the baton and crossing the finish line with me. Thank you for the fierce, elegant, and determined energy you gave this book right when it needed it. Anything with Selena! Selena, you carried us when it felt like everything was falling apart. Thank you for breathing more life into the bones of this precious book. You protected and honored my words and made them shine. Wendy, thank you for saying yes and paving way for this book and for me. Richelle, you were my prenatal vitamins and gave me all I needed to make this book a reality. You sprinkled your magic fairy dust and helped me believe in me. Thank you. Ana Flores, my OG fairygodmother, you were the one who started it all. Gracias will never be enough.

I want to thank my community. Thank you to the Badass x Bonita community who surrounded me when I felt most alone. Thank you for walking with me as we collectively learn to love ourselves. Gracias a mis Mujeres Mariposas. Es un honor verlas volar. Thank you to all my Queer Girls Around the World. Queer girls do it better. Gracias a los de Ranchito con Esperanza where I became Ms. Kim Possible, y a los Bailadores de Bronce, for being my refuge and connecting me to mi cultura in Seattle. Sending love to those from Chi Alpha at Cornell for loving me when you did. Gracias a todos los que me acercaron a Dios.

Gracias a Roo, mi angelito gay de la CDMX. Te amo y estoy agradecida por tu ser, apoyo, consejos, las recogidas al aeropuerto, las noches que me dejaste quedarme contigo y Paprika, todo. Gracias a Fede, mi mejor amigo, compañero del alma Edwin Soto Saucedo. Love you un chingo y medio. Siempre.

Amado mío, gracias por ser y dejarme ser. Gracias por tu amor puro y de fuego. Mi alma bonita, *il amore della mia vita*. Gracias por cuidarme, por todas las pastas, las risas, las lágrimas y nuestras aventuras. *Piano, piano*, lo estamos logrando. Todo mi corazón tiene tu nombre escrito. Por ti conozco el amor más puro y profundo. Contigo estoy escribiendo la historia de amor más bella. *Ti amo*.

NOTES

CHAPTER 1

1. Betty Friedan, *The Feminine Mystique* (New York: W. W. Norton & Company, 2001), 22.
2. Giovanna De Oliveira, et al., "Social Determinants of Depression Among Hispanic Women," *Journal of the American Psychiatric Nurses Association,* 23, no. 1 (September 19, 2016): 28–36, https://doi.org/10.1177 /1078390316669230.
3. William E. Cross, Linda C. Strauss, and Peony E. Fhagen-Smith, "African American Identity Development Across the Life Span: Educational Implications," in *Routledge eBooks,* 1999, 39–58, https://doi.org/10.4324 /9781410601568-7.
4. Audre Lorde, *Sister Outsider: Essays and Speeches* (New York: Ten Speed Press, 1984), 42, http://ci.nii.ac.jp/ncid/BA01234259.
5. Kotkin, Joel, and Erika Ozuna. "The Changing Face of the San Fernando Valley." *Pepperdine University Public Policy,* 2002: 13–14. https:/ /publicpolicy.pepperdine.edu/davenport-institute/content/reports /changing-face.pdf.
6. Teresa De Lauretis, "Queer Theory: Lesbian and Gay Sexualities, an Introduction," *Differences,* 3, no. 2 (Summer 1991): iii–xviii, https://doi.org /10.1215/10407391-3-2-iii.
7. Gracia Trujillo, *El Feminismo Queer Es Para Todo El Mundo* (Madrid: Catarata, 2022), 16.
8. Gracia Trujillo, *El Feminismo Queer Es Para Todo El Mundo* (Madrid: Catarata, 2022) 16.
9. Gracia Trujillo, *El Feminismo Queer Es Para Todo El Mundo* (Madrid: Catarata, 2022) 24.
10. Gracia Trujillo, *El Feminismo Queer Es Para Todo El Mundo* (Madrid: Catarata, 2022) 24.
11. Gracia Trujillo, *El Feminismo Queer Es Para Todo El Mundo* (Madrid: Catarata, 2022) 19.
12. Michael Warner, "Fear of a Queer Planet: Queer Politics and Social Theory," *Contemporary Sociology,* 23, no. 6 (November 1, 1994): xxi, https://doi.org /10.2307/2076123.

13. Lisa Duggan, "The New Homonormativity: The Sexual Politics of Neoliberalism." *Duke University Press eBooks* (May 2020): 179, https://doi.org/10.1515/9780822383901-008.
14. Audre Lorde, *Sister Outsider: Essays and Speeches* (New York: Ten Speed Press, 1984), 41, http://ci.nii.ac.jp/ncid/BA01234259.

CHAPTER 2

1. Galit Atlas, *Emotional Inheritance: Moving beyond the legacy of trauma* (Boston: Little, Brown Spark, 2022).
2. Rachael A. Dansby and Jason B. Whiting, "Second-Order Change in Couple and Family Therapy." Encyclopedia of Couple and Family Therapy (2017): 1–4, https://doi.org/10.1007/978-3-319-15877-8_307-1.
3. Diksha Kashyap, "Essay on Personality: Meaning, Nature and Determinants." Your Article Library. (September 30, 2015), https://www.yourarticlelibrary.com/essay/personality-essay/essay-on-personality-meaning-nature-and-determinants/63789.
4. "Adverse Childhood Experiences (ACEs)." The Burke Foundation (n.d.), https://burkefoundation.org/what-drives-us/adverse-childhood-experiences-aces/.
5. "Adverse Childhood Experiences (ACEs)." The Burke Foundation (n.d.), https://burkefoundation.org/what-drives-us/adverse-childhood-experiences-aces/.
6. Priscilla, Leslie. "The Madre Wound: What It Is, and How to Heal It." Scary Mommy, September 14, 2021. https://www.scarymommy.com/madre-wound-what-it-is-and-how-to-heal-it.
7. Perpetua Neo, "12 Signs You Grew up With a Narcissistic Mother & How It May Affect You Today," Mindbodygreen, June 6, 2023, https://www.mindbodygreen.com/articles/narcissistic-mother.
8. Ibid.

CHAPTER 3

1. Cachelin FM, Gil-Rivas V, Vela A. Understanding Eating Disorders among Latinas. *Adv Eat Disord.* 2014 Jan 1;2(2):204–208. doi: 10.1080/21662630.2013.869391. PMID: 24999448; PMCID: PMC4078895.
2. Melody Beattie, *Codependent No More: How to Stop Controlling Others and Start Caring for Yourself* (Center City, Minn.: Hazelden Publishing, 1986): 35–36, http://ci.nii.ac.jp/ncid/BA73592298.
3. Melody Beattie, *Codependent No More: How to Stop Controlling Others and Start Caring for Yourself* (Center City, Minn.: Hazelden Publishing, 1986): 42-52, http://ci.nii.ac.jp/ncid/BA73592298.
4. Bell Hooks, *All About Love: New Visions* (New York: Perennial, 2000): 10, https://ci.nii.ac.jp/ncid/BA52796948.

5. "Mexico Records Alarming Figures for Child Sexual Abuse in Latin America." *Yo Digo No Más* (blog), July 31, 2023. https://yodigonomas .com/en/blog/mexico-records-alarming-figures-for-child-sexual-abuse-in -latin-america/.

6. Gloria González-López, *Secretos de familia: Incesto y violencia sexual en México* (Coyoacán, México: Siglo XXI Editores México, 2019), 27.

7. Vazquez, Maria. "Silencing the self, relationship satisfaction and marianismo: An analysis of depression of Latinas." *Dissertation Abstracts International: Section B: The Sciences and Engineering*, 59, no. (4-B) (1998):1871. https: //psycnet.apa.org/record/1998-95020-230.

8. FederalSafetyNet.com. "U.S. Poverty Statistics" Federal Safety Net (March 1, 2024), https://federalsafetynet.com/poverty-statistics/.

9. Torres, Jannesse, and Lianne Torres. "2 Sisters, 2 Survivors." Acast, Spotify. October 26, 2022. Accessed March 1, 2024. https://open.spotify.com /episode/1tuqPiLaxMyJ0dRxbgqUYN?si=h2TKG1I6Q6CMEDyd MKKk3g.

10. Smith, Brendan L. "Spanish-speaking Psychologists in Demand." Monitor on Psychology (June 2018), 68, https://www.apa.org/monitor/2018/06 /spanish-speaking#:~:text=In%20a%20nationwide%20APA %20survey,limit%20access%20to%20quality%20care.

11. Chen, Yiyu, and María A. Ramos-Olazagasti. "Over One Third of Lower-income Latino Adults Living with Children Have Frequent Anxiety or Depressive Symptoms, and Most Do Not Receive Mental Health Services." National Research Center on Hispanic Children & Families (July 19, 2022), https://doi.org/10.59377/244k3083b.

CHAPTER 4

1. Blanco, Margarita. *Sanación emocional del niño interior: Método Ser Mejor Ser*, 2014, Publicaciones Vedra S.L., 25-26.

2. Brown, Daniel P., and David S. Elliott. *Attachment Disturbances in Adults: Treatment for Comprehensive Repair*. (New York: W. W. Norton & Company, 2016, pages 75–78).

3. APA Dictionary of Psychology. American Psychological Association (updated April 19, 2018), https://dictionary.apa.org/attunement.

CHAPTER 5

1. "Building Trauma-Informed Communities." Public Health Matters Blog, CDC, May 25, 2022. https://blogs.cdc.gov/publichealthmatters/2022/05 /trauma-informed/#:~:text=Trauma%20is%20a%20physical%2C %20cognitive,lasting%20effects%2C%20particularly%20if%20untreated.

2. Bubrick, Jerry, PhD. "Signs of Trauma in Children." Child Mind Institute, October 30, 2023. https://childmind.org/article/signs-trauma-children /#:~:text=The%20signs%20of%20trauma%20in%20a%20child

%20include%20obsession%20with,the%20death%20of%20a %20classmate.

3. "Adverse Childhood Experiences (ACEs)." The Burke Foundation, n.d. https://burkefoundation.org/what-drives-us/adverse-childhood -experiences-aces/.

4. Ellen Bass and Laura Davis, *The Courage to Heal 4e: A Guide for Women Survivors of Child Sexual Abuse 20th Anniversary Edition* (New York: Harper Collins, 2008), 3.

5. Ellen Bass and Laura Davis, *The Courage to Heal 4e: A Guide for Women Survivors of Child Sexual Abuse 20th Anniversary Edition* (New York: Harper Collins, 2008), 5–7.

6. Ellen Bass and Laura Davis, *The Courage to Heal 4e: A Guide for Women Survivors of Child Sexual Abuse 20th Anniversary Edition* (New York: Harper Collins, 2008), 242–245.

7. "PTSD and DSM-5." National Center for PTSD. U.S. Department of Veterans Affairs   (n.d.), https://www.ptsd.va.gov/professional/treat /essentials/dsm5_ptsd.asp.

8. Ellen Bass and Laura Davis, *The Courage to Heal 4e: A Guide for Women Survivors of Child Sexual Abuse 20th Anniversary Edition* (New York: Harper Collins, 2008), 244.

9. Martin E. P. Seligman, "Learned Helplessness," *Annual Review of Medicine*, 23, no. 1 (February 1, 1972): 407–12, https://doi.org/10.1146/annurev .me.23.020172.002203.

CHAPTER 6

1. Amir Levine and Rachel S. F. Heller, *Attached: The New Science of Adult Attachment and How It Can Help You Find—and Keep—Love* (London: TarcherPerigee, 2012).

2. Milan Yerkovich and Kay Yerkovich, *How We Love, Expanded Edition: Discover Your Love Style, Enhance Your Marriage* (New York: WaterBrook, 2009).

3. Milan Yerkovich and Kay Yerkovich, *How We Love, Expanded Edition: Discover Your Love Style, Enhance Your Marriage* (New York: WaterBrook, 2009).

4. Milan Yerkovich and Kay Yerkovich, *How We Love, Expanded Edition: Discover Your Love Style, Enhance Your Marriage* (New York: WaterBrook, 2009).

CHAPTER 8

1. Ada María Isasi-Díaz, *Mujerista Theology: A Theology for the Twenty-First Century* (Maryknoll, New York: Orbis Books, 1996) 60, http://ci.nii.ac.jp /ncid/BA45036092.

2. Ada María Isasi-Díaz, *Mujerista Theology: A Theology for the Twenty-First Century* (Maryknoll, New York: Orbis Books, 1996), 25, http://ci.nii.ac.jp /ncid/BA45036092.
3. Betty Friedan, *The Feminine Mystique* (New York: W. W. Norton & Company, 2001), 93.
4. Betty Friedan, *The Feminine Mystique* (New York: W. W. Norton & Company, 2001), 34.

CHAPTER 10
1. Nedra Glover Tawwab, *Set Boundaries, Find Peace: A Guide to Reclaiming Yourself* (London: TarcherPerigee, 2021, pages 9–12).

CHAPTER 12
1. Indigo Staff, "Chavela Vargas: una vida a contracorriente," Reporte Indigo, September 18, 2017, https://www.reporteindigo.com/piensa/chavela-vargas -perfil-vida-contracorriente-aniversario-muerte-musica-ranchera/.

ABOUT THE AUTHOR

Kim Guerra is a queer woman of color. A butterfly woman who has given herself wings. She is a writer, therapist, and creator. Guerra is the creator of *Badass x Bonita, Queer Girl Around the World*, and *Queer Art Around the World*, projects she considers to be a work of art, self-love, and community liberation. She was born and raised in the San Fernando Valley in Los Angeles. Kim graduated from Cornell University and received her master's in Marriage and Family Therapy from Antioch University in Seattle. Her heart is rooted in Mexico and her wings take her around the world.